Series Editor

Michael J. Parnham
PLIVA
Research Institute
Prilaz baruna Filipovica 25
1000 Zagreb
Croatia

Chemokines and Skin

E. Kownatzki
J. Norgauer

Editors

Springer Basel AG

Editors

Prof. Dr. Eckhard Kownatzki
Dr. Johannes Norgauer
Abteilung für Experimentelle Dermatologie
Klinikum der Albert-Ludwigs-Universität
Hauptstr. 7
D-79104 Freiburg
Germany

Library of Congress Cataloging-in-Publication Data
Chemokines and skin / edited by Eckhard Kownatzki, Johannes Norgauer.
     p.   cm. -- (PIR – Progress in inflammation research)
   Includes bibliographical references and index.
   ISBN 978-3-0348-9797-6   ISBN 978-3-0348-8843-1 (eBook)
   DOI 10.1007/978-3-0348-8843-1
   1. Chemokines.   2. Skin--Inflammation.   3. Skin--Immunology.
 I. Kownatzki, Eckhard.   II. Norgauer, Johannes.   III. Series: PIR (Series)
 QR185.8j.C45C48   1998
 616.07'9--dc21
 98-18186
 CIP

Deutsche Bibliothek Cataloging-in-Publication Data
Chemokines and Skin / ed. by Eckhard Kownatzki ;
Johannes Norgauer. - Basel ; Boston ; Berlin : Birkhäuser, 1998
   (Progress in inflammation research)
   ISBN 978-3-0348-9797-6

© 1998 Springer Basel AG
Originally published by Birkhäuser Verlag, Basel, Switzerland in 1998
Softcover reprint of the hardcover 1st edition 1998

Printed on acid-free paper produced from chlorine-free pulp. TCF ∞
Cover design: Markus Etterich, Basel

ISBN 978-3-0348-9797-6

9 8 7 6 5 4 3 2 1

Contents

List of contributors

Paola Allavena, Istituto di Ricerche Farmacologiche "Mario Negri", Via Eritrea 62, I-20157 Milan, Italy; e-mail: Allavena@irfmn.mnegri.it

Delia Bussfeld, Institute of Immunology, Philipps-University Marburg, Robert-Koch-Str. 17, D-35037 Marburg, Germany

Eva Engelhardt, Department of Dermatology, University of Würzburg Medical School, Josef-Schneider-Str. 2, D-97080 Würzburg, Germany

Diethard Gemsa, Institute of Immunology, Philipps-University Marburg, Robert-Koch-Str. 17, D-35037 Marburg, Germany

Reinhard Gillitzer, Department of Dermatology, University of Würzburg Medical School, Josef-Schneider-Str. 2, D-97080 Würzburg, Germany;
e-mail: gillitzer-r.derma@mail.uni-wuerzburg, Germany

Matthias Goebeler, Department of Dermatology, University of Würzburg Medical School, Josef-Schneider-Str. 2, D-97080 Würzburg, Germany

Andreas Grützkau, Department of Dermatology, Charité-Virchow Clinic, Humboldt University, Augustenburger Platz 1, D-13344 Berlin, Germany;
e-mail: a-gtzkau@ukru.de

Beate M. Henz, Department of Dermatology, Charité-Virchow Clinic, Augustenburger Platz 1, D-13344 Berlin, Germany; e-mail: mfuchs@ukru.de

Robert C. Hoch, Department of Immunology, The Scripps Research Institute, 10550 N. Torrey Pines Rd., La Jolla, CA 92037, USA; e-mail: rhoch@scripps.edu

Clemens Hofmann, Department of Experimental Dermatology, University of Freiburg, Hauptstr. 7, D-79104 Freiburg, Germany;
e-mail: Hofmann@haut.ukl.uni-freiburg.de

Tan Jinquan, Department of Immunology, Anhui Medical University, 69 Meishan Road, Hefai 230032, Anhui Province, People's Republic of China

Andreas Kaufmann, Institute of Immunology, Philipps-University Marburg, Robert-Koch-Str. 17, D-35037 Marburg, Germany

Sabine Krüger-Krasagakes, Department of Dermatology, Charité-Virchow Clinic, Humboldt University, Augustenburger Platz 1, D-13344 Berlin, Germany

Undine Lippert, Department of Dermatology, University Hospital, von-Siebold-Strasse 3, D-37075 Göttingen, Germany; e-mail: ulipper@gwdg.de

Alberto Mantovani, Istituto di Ricerche Farmacologiche Mario Negri, Via Eritrea 62, I-20157 Milan, Italy; and Department of Biotechnology, Section of General Pathology, University of Brescia, Italy; e-mail: Mantovani@irfmn.mnegri.it

Beatrix Metzner, Department of Experimental Dermatology, University of Freiburg, Hauptstr. 7, D-79104 Freiburg, Germany

Johannes Norgauer, Department of Experimental Dermatology, University of Freiburg, Hauptstr. 7, D-79104 Freiburg, Germany;
e-mail: norgauer@haut.ukl.uni-freiburg-de

Frank Peters, Department of Experimental Dermatology, University of Freiburg, Hauptstr. 7, D-79104 Freiburg, Germany

Ingrid U. Schraufstätter, Department of Immunology, The Scripps Research Institute, 10550 N. Torrey Pines Rd., La Jolla, CA 92037, USA;
e-mail: ingridsc@scripps.edu

Jens-M. Schröder, Department of Dermatology, University of Kiel, Schittenhelm-str.7, D-24105 Kiel, Germany; e-mail: jschroeder@dermatology.uni-kiel.de

Silvano Sozzani, Istituto di Ricerche Farmacologiche "Mario Negri", Via Eritrea 62, I-20157 Milan, Italy; e-mail: Sozzani@irfmn.mnegri.it

Hans Sprenger, Institute of Laboratory Medicine, Leopoldina-Hospital, Gustav-Adolf-Str. 8, D-97422 Schweinfurt, Germany

Hiroshi Takamori, Department of Surgery, Kumamoto University, Kumamoto 860, Japan; e-mail: kei@kaiju.medic.Kumamoto-u.ac.jp

Kristian Thestrup-Pedersen, Department of Dermatology, Marselisborg Hospital, University of Aarhus, DK-8000 Aarhus, Denmark;
e-mail: akh.grp03s.ktp@aaa.dk

Ulrich Zimpfer, Department of Experimental Dermatology, University of Freiburg, Hauptstr. 7, D-79104 Freiburg, Germany;
 e-mail: zimpfer@haut.ukl.uni-freiburg.de

Introduction

The accumulation of white blood cells is a hallmark of inflammation. The penetration through the vessel walls and the infiltration around the inflammatory stimulus is a complex process which involves active adherence and directed migration of the inflammatory cells. Chemotactic factors stimulate both adherence and migration. Technical tools such as the Boyden chamber [1] made it possible to study leukocyte migration *in vitro*. This technique allows differentiation between migration directed towards a chemotactic stimulus and non-directed migration.

Until a decade ago only two naturally occurring molecules had been clearly identified as potent chemotactic attractants of neutrophilic granulocytes. They were the split product of the fifth complement component C5a [2] and the arachidonic acid metabolite leukotriene B_4 [3]. In 1986, a novel human monocyte-derived chemotaxin attracting neutrophilic granulocytes with a similar potency was found [4]. This report was quickly confirmed by several groups [5–8]. The new factor was purified, cloned and sequenced [9, 10]. The term "interleukin 8" (IL-8) replaced the various names proposed previously [4–8].

Sequence data revealed that IL-8 belonged to a large family of chemotactic cytokines, now called "chemokines" [11]. Four subfamilies were distinguished on the basis of the number and position of the first cysteine residues. They are designated accordingly as C, CC, CXC and CX_3C chemokines [11–13]. The number of human chemokines identified so far is close to 40 [11–13].

Chemokines direct the trafficking, not only of granulocytes and monocytes, but they also attract lymphocytes and appear to be responsible for lymphocyte recruitment [11]. Chemokine activities not immediately associated with inflammatory reactions include the proliferation of transformed cells as well as angiogenic and angiostatic effects. Of great current interest is the function of chemokine receptors as cofactors for the entry of HIV [14, 15].

The skin is an obvious site of inflammatory reactions. About half of all skin diseases requiring the attention of a dermatologist are of inflammatory nature. The easy accessibility makes the skin suitable for analyzing mechanisms of inflammation in general and the involvement of chemokines in particular. Such an analysis should be of both theoretical and practical value.

For the present volume, we have asked several authors actively engaged in the field to review what is currently known about chemokines and their relevance for skin inflammation and skin diseases. The first three chapters deal with the structure and molecular biology of chemokines and their receptors. The following three chapters review information on the interaction of chemokines with lymphocytes, mast cells and eosinophilic granulocytes. One chapter describes the involvement of chemokines in several inflammatory skin diseases. The final chapter reports on *in vitro* evidence for a growth-promotion of skin-derived tumor cells by chemokines.

The volume summarizes the present state of knowledge concerning chemokines. Progress in the field is still moving at a fast pace. It is likely that more members of the various subfamilies will be discovered and possibly even new subfamilies. More cells will be identified as both sources and targets of chemokines, and additional functional activities will be attributable to these molecules. A few unusual features are already apparent with the present information. Compared with the "classical" cytokines such as IL-1, TNFα, IFNγ and GM-CSF, chemokines appear to have a limited number of activities on cells, mostly related to inflammation and above all to cell migration. On the other hand, there is a large number of different chemokines and of variants of single chemokines. Thereby it is possible to specifically obtain a desirable result with a single molecule or a combination of a small number of molecules. For the observer such events may be easier to understand than the blinding complexity so often encountered when dealing with cytokines and their interactions.

Freiburg, December 1997

Eckhard Kownatzki
Johannes Norgauer

References

1   Boyden S (1962) The chemotactic activity of mixtures of antibody and antigen on polymorphonuclear leucocytes. *J Exp Med* 115: 453–466
2   Hugli TE (1981) The structural basis for anaphylatoxin and chemotactic functions of C3a, C4a and C5a. *Crit Rev Immunol* 1: 321–366
3   Ford-Hutchinson AW, Bray MA, Doig MV, Shipley ME, Smith MJH (1980) Leukotriene B$_4$, a potent chemokinetic and aggregating substance released from polymorphonuclear leukocytes. *Nature* 286: 264–265
4   Kownatzki E, Kapp A, Uhrich S (1986) Novel neutrophil chemotactic factor derived from human peripheral blood mononuclear leucocytes. *Clin Exp Immunol* 64: 214–222
5   Yoshimura TK, Matsushima K, Oppenheim JJ, Leonard EJ (1987) Neutrophil chemotactic factor produced by lipopolysaccharide (LPS)-stimulated human blood mononu-

clear leukocytes: Partial characterization and separation from interleukin 1 (IL-1). *J Immunol* 139: 788–793

6   Schroeder JM, Mrowietz U, Morita E, Christophers E (1987) Purification and partial biochemical characterization of a human monocyte-derived neutrophilactivating peptide that lacks interleukin 1 activity. *J Immunol* 139: 3474–3483

7   Walz A, Peveri P, Aschauer H, Baggiolini M (1987) Purification and amino acid sequencing of NAF, a novel neutrophil-activating factor produced by monocytes. *Biochem Biophys Res Commun* 151: 883–889

8   Van Damme J, Van Beeumen J, Opdenakker G, Billiau A (1988) A novel, NH_2-terminal sequence-characterized human monokine possessing neutrophil chemotactic, skin-reactive, and granulocytosis-promoting activity. *J Exp Med* 167: 1364–1376

9   Lindley I, Aschauer H, Seifert JM, Lam C, Brunowsky W, Kownatzki E, Thelen M, Peveri P, Dewald B, von Tscharner V et al (1988) Synthesis and expression in *Escherichia coli* of the gene encoding monocyte-derived neutrophil-activating factor: Biological equivalence between natural and recombinant neutrophil-activating factor. *Proc Natl Acad Sci USA* 85: 9199–9203

10   Matsushima K, Morishita K, Yoshimura T (1988) Molecular cloning of cDNA from a human monocyte derived neutrophil chemotactic factor (MDNCF) and the induction of MDNCF mRNA by interleukin-1 and tumor necrosis factor. *J Exp Med* 167: 1883–1898J

11   Baggiolini M, Dewald B, Moser B (1997) Human chemokines: An update. *Ann Rev Immunol* 15: 675–705

12   Bazan JF, Bacon KB, Hardiman WW, Soo K, Rossi D, Greaves DR, Zlotnik A, Schall TJ (1997) A new class of membrane-bound chemokine with a CX_3C motif. *Nature* 385: 640–644

13   Pan Y, Lloyd C, Zhou H, Dolich S, Deeds J, Gonzalo JA, Vath J, Gosselin M, Ma J, Dussault B et al (1997) Neurotactin, a membrane-anchored chemokine upregulated in brain inflammation. *Nature* 387: 611–617

14   Fauci AS (1996) Host factors and the pathogenesis of HlV-induced disease. *Nature* 384: 529–534

15   He J, Chen Y, Farzan M, Choe H, Ohagen A, Gartner S, Busciglio J, Yang X, Hofmann W, Newman W et al (1997) CCR3 and CCR5 are co-receptors for HIV1 infection of microglia. *Nature* 385: 645–649

Chemokines: Attraction of dendritic cells and role in tumor immunobiology

Alberto Mantovani[1], Paola Allavena and Silvano Sozzani

Istituto di Ricerche Farmacologiche "Mario Negri", Via Eritrea 62, 20157 Milan, Italy;
[1] also at the Dept. of Biotechnology, Section of General Pathology, University of Brescia, Italy

Introduction

In this chapter we will discuss selected aspects of the structure and function of chemokines, with emphasis on monocyte chemotactic proteins (MCPs) as prototypic CC chemokine. Among functions, we will emphasize recent results on molecules which attract dendritic cells of obvious relevance for skin immunobiology and emphasize potential relevance for tumor therapy.

Several independent lines of work lead to the identification of monocyte chemotactic protein-1 (MCP-1) and related molecules. Already in the early 1970s it had been noted that supernatants of activated blood mononuclear cells contained attractants active on monocytes and neutrophils [1]. Subsequently, a chemotactic factor active on monocytes was identified in culture supernatants of mouse [2] and human [3, 4] tumor lines and called tumor-derived chemotactic factor (TDCF) [3–5]. TDCF was at the time rather unique in that it was active on monocytes but not on neutrophils [4] and had a low (12kDa) molecular weight [3, 4]. Moreover, correlative evidence suggested its involvement in the regulation of macrophage infiltration in murine and human tumors [3, 4, 6]. A molecule with similar cellular specificity and physicochemical properties was independently identified in the culture supernatant of smooth muscle cells (SMDCF) [7]. The JE gene had been identified as an immediate-early PDGF-inducible gene in fibroblasts [8, 9]. Thus, in the mid 1980s a gene (JE) was in search of a function, and a monocyte-specific attractant was awaiting molecular definition. In 1989, MCP-1 was successfully purified from supernatants of a human glioma [10] a human monocytic leukemia [11] and a human sarcoma [12– 14]: sequencing and molecular cloning revealed its relationship with the long known JE gene [15–17].

Structural consideration

The presence of conserved Cys (4 or 2) residues defines chemokine families characterized by a CC, CXC, C or CX3C motif [18]. CXC chemokines attract mainly neu-

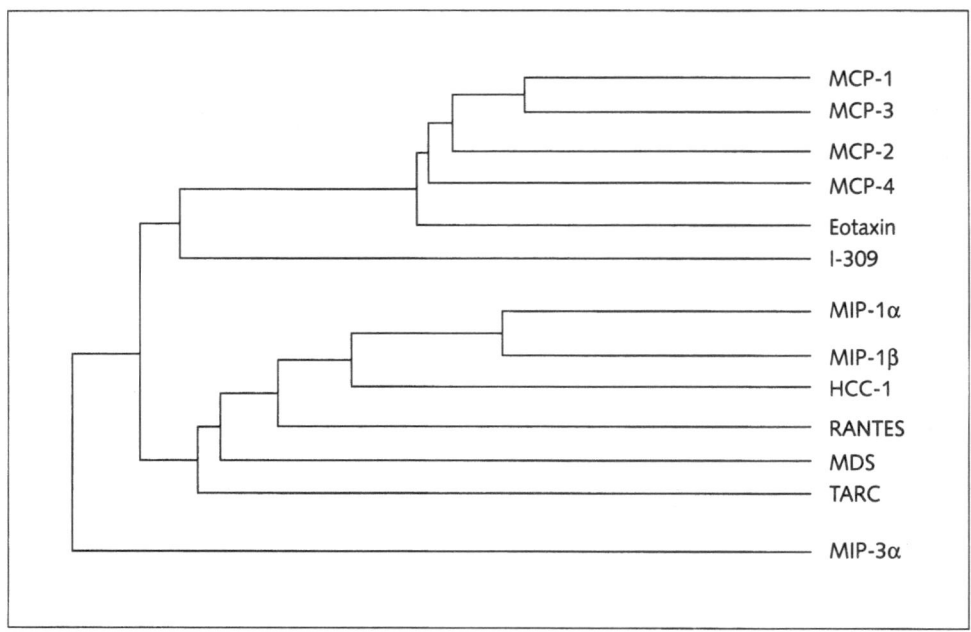

Figure 1
Dendrogram analysis of CC chemokines

trophils and T lymphocytes, whereas other molecules have a broader spectrum of action. The presence or absence of an ELR motif preceding CXC defines whether CXC chemokines are active (e.g. IL-8) or inactive (e.g. IP-10) on neutrophils. ELR-chemokines are active on T cells. CC chemokines share other sequence similarities such as a C-terminal helix and hydropholic sequences in the first and third β sheet.

Dendrogram analysis (Fig. 1) reveals that chemokines can be grouped. For instance, all MCPs and eotaxin are related, whereas one group includes the Macrophage Inflammatory Proteins (MIPs), including viral MIP encoded by human herpes virus-8 involved in the pathogenesis of Kaposi's sarcoma, and RANTES.

Chemokines are localized at distinct chromosomal regions (Tab. 1). Most CC chemokines are localized on chromosome 17, in two clusters (MCPs and MIP/RANTES) which reflect sequence similarity. However, some recently identified chemokines show a distinct chromosomal localization. Macrophage derived chemokine (MDC), Thymus Activation-Regulated Chemokine (TARC) and fraktalkine are localized on chromosome 16, and ELC and MIP-3α/LARC are on chromosome 9 and 2, respectively [18–22].

The structural properties of MCP-1 and related molecules will now be discussed in more detail.

Table 1
Chromosomal localization of chemokines (human)

	Chromosome	Chemokines
CC	17q11 - 921	MCPs, MIPs/RANTES
	16 q	MDC, TARC
	9 q	MIP3β, SLC
	2 q	LARC
C	1	Lymphotactin
CX3C	16	Fractalkine
CXC	2	IL-8, GRO_s

Protein and gene structure

Human MCP-1 is a glycoprotein of 76 residues with four cysteines forming two intramolecular disulfide bridges [15–17, 23]. Using a combination of sequencing of proteolytic fragments and mass spectrometry, the complete amino acid sequence of human MCP-1 could be determined [24]. Except for some minor amino-terminal processed forms [25, 26], the amino-terminus of mature MCP-1 protein is blocked for Edman degradation by a pyroglutamic acid residue. One N-glycosylation site is located close to the amino-terminus and several glycosylated forms of MCP-1 have been reported ranging from 9 kDa to 17 kDa on SDS-PAGE. The addition of O-linked sugar and sialic acid residue contributes to the different molecular weight forms of MCP-1 [10, 24, 25, 27]. MCP-1 is a basic protein (pI = 10.6) that shows affinity for heparin.

MNR studies on the solution structure of IL-8 and MIP-1β revealed a number of structural differences between CC and CXC chemokines [28, 29]. IL-8 was found to be globular in shape, whereas for MIP-1β a more cylindrical structure is proposed. In contrast to the IL-8 α-helices, both MIP-1β a-helices were found to be located at opposite sites of the molecule. Thus, the MIP-1β monomer structure is similar to the IL-8 structure but the interface and quaternary structure are completely different. Recent studies using size exclusion HPLC, sedimentation equilibrium and chemical cross-linking have shown that, at physiological (low nanomolar) concentrations, MCP-1 as well as IL-8 and I-309 occur as monomer instead of dimers [30]. MCP-1, as well as IL-8, forms an equilibrium between the monomeric and dimeric form. At concentrations above 100 μM almost all MCP-1 is the dimeric condition, but at physiologically active concentrations (<100 nM) MCP-1 nearly exclusively occurs as monomer.

Natural MCP-2 and -3 proteins were copurified from conditioned medium of osteosarcoma cells and identified by amino acid sequence analysis [31]. MCP-2 and MCP-3 contain 76 amino acids, including four cysteines which are characteristic for the chemokine family. Both peptides display high sequence similarity to MCP-1 (62% and 71% identity, respectively). MCP-2 and MCP-3 are slightly more basic than MCP-1 (pI = 10.6) with theoretical pI's of 10.9, respectively. Similar to all other animal MCPs isolated so far, human MCP-2 and MCP-3 also appeared to be blocked at the amino-terminus so that protein sequence data were obtained by Edman degradation of proteolytic fragments [31]. The MCP-2 sequence does not contain N-glycosylation sites. Based upon the theoretical relative molecular mass (8893 Da) and on the apparent molecular weight of 7.5 kDa on SDS-PAGE [31, 32], no O-glycosylation is to be expected for MCP-2. Natural human MCP-3 occurred as an 11 kDa protein on SDS-PAGE [31]. Although the cDNA derived protein sequence contains one amino-terminally located N-glycosylation site [33, 34], natural 11 kDa MCP-3 did not appear to be N-glycosylated [35]. Moreover, folded synthetic MCP-3 also appeared as an 11 kDa protein on SDS-PAGE, although the theoretical relative molecular mass is only 8935 Da [32]. In addition to the unglycosylated MCP-3 form [33], multiple forms (11, 13, 17 and 18 kDa) were detected after expression in COS cells. Here, both N- and O-glycosylation were involved. Electrospray mass spectrometry (MS) of the unglycosylated protein confirmed the amino-terminal pyroglutamate and the existence of two disulfide bridges.

The MCP-1, MIP-2 and MCP-3 genes with the locus symbols SCYA2, SCYA8 and SCYA7 (small inducible cytokine genes number 2, 8 and 7), respectively, were assigned to the CC chemokine gene cluster on human chromosome 17q11.2-12 [35–38].

The MCP-1 gene consists of three exons and two introns [39, 40]. The translated MCP-1 mRNA codes for a 99 amino acid precursor protein including a 23 amino acids long, mainly hydrophobic leader sequence. The promoter region contains the TATA box, 96 bp upstream of the translation initiation site. The polyadenylation site (AATAA) is located 353 bp downstream of the stop codon. The GGAAGATC-CCT consensus sequence for the kB enhancer element (position -148), which is possibly involved in lipopolysaccharide (LPS) and tumor necrosis factor (TNF) responses, and the ATTTGCGT consensus sequence for the octamer transcription factor (OTF at position -282) were found further in the promoter region [40]. In addition to a GC-box (at -126 bp), two TPA-responsive elements (TRE) for the binding of transacting factor AP-1 (TGACTCC and TCACTCA) are found at positions -128 and -156, respectively. Several other kB binding sites and TREs were discovered in the enhancer region, between 2 and 3 kbp upstream from the translation initiation site [41]. Promoter and enhancer regions thus contain cis-elements which are possibly important for the regulation of MCP-1 gene transcription. The two cis-elements, essential for the MCP-1 induction and for the maintenance of basal MCP-1 transcriptional activity, were found to be the Sp-1 binding GC-box at position -126 in the promoter region and the kB binding site at position -2672 in the enhancer region, respectively. All other kB binding sites and TREs are to be nonfunctional. The essential nuclear factor-kb (NF-kB) and Sp-1 binding sites cannot, however, completely explain the MCP-1 gene transcription since, for example, in lymphocytes virtually no MCP-1 mRNA is found [42], although the Sp-1 expression is rather high [41].

Much like for the MCP-1 gene, three exons and two introns are included in the MCP-3 gene. Similar to the MCP-1 exons, the MCP-3 exons encode a protein of 99 residues, which includes a 23 amino acid signal sequence. The promoter region of the MCP-3 gene contains two tandem dinucleotide repeats (TDR), (CA)17 and (GA)7, a property which is shared with the MIP-1α and I-309 gene sequences. Direct and indirect repeats (DR and IR) as well as palindromic sequences (Pal), which might enhance DNA recombinatorial events, are also clustered in this region. Other interesting features like the CAAT-box, the TATA-box, a Cap-signal, the transcription initiation site and at the 3' end a mRNA hairpin loop, an AT-rich mRNA destabilizing region and the polyadenylation site are described by [35].

The murine equivalent of human MCP-1 has been identified as the competence gene JE, regulated by PDGF [8, 43]. Surprisingly the JE gene codes for an NH2-terminally blocked protein with an additional COOH-terminal tail (49 amino acids) compared to human MCP-1. The corresponding biologically active protein has been isolated from virally infected fibroblasts [44]. The murine homologue of MCP-3 has been isolated from macrophages using a cDNA probe for human MCP-3 [45]. The sequence was found to be identical to that of MARC, derived from mast cells challenged with immunoglobulin E and antigen [46] and FIC isolated from fibroblasts stimulated with serum [47]. Mouse JE and MARC show 55% and 59% amino acid sequence similarity with human MCP-1 and MCP-3, respectively [34].

Tumors as a paradigm for chemokines: Recruitment

Rather than reviewing actions of chemokines on different leukocyte populations, which will be discussed elsewhere in this book, here we will summarize the involvement of these molecules in the immunobiology of neoplastic tissues. We propose that tumors provide a paradigm for the *in vivo* function of chemokines. In addition, emerging evidence on the action of chemokines on dendritic cells, of obvious relevance in the context of this book, will be discussed.

Murine tumors

The percentage of TAM for each tumor is usually maintained as a relatively stable "individual" property during tumor growth and upon transplantation in syngeneic hosts. Transplantation of xenogeneic human (but not allogeneic murine) tumors is associated with a different pattern of distribution, peripheral versus diffuse, of TAM within the lesion [48]. Macrophages also infiltrate metastatic lesions, although TAM have been less extensively studied in secondary foci [6]. Even at macrophage-rich anatomical sites such as the liver, macrophage infiltration in metastasis depends to a large extent upon recruitment of monocytic precursors [49]. Experiments in which tumors were transplanted in hosts with defective T- or natural killer cell immunity suggest that, for many neoplasms, specific immunity is not a major determinant of macrophage infiltration, and that factors derived from the tumor itself play a pivotal role in the regulation of macrophage levels in poorly immunogenic metastatic tumors [6].

Analysis of mechanisms of recruitment of macrophages in tumors was one pathway that led to the identification of MCP-1 [3, 6, 10, 14, 50]. Several lines of evidence suggest that MCP-1 can represent an important determinant of the levels of TAM [6, 51]. In early studies with murine tumors or human tumors in nude mice a correlation was found between MCP-1 activity and percentage of TAM, a finding confirmed in subsequent experiments with the MCP-1 probe [51]. Subcutaneous inoculation of tumor-derived human MCP-1, MCP-2 and MCP-3 led to macrophage infiltration [12, 31, 52]. Finally, and conclusively, transfer of the mouse or human MCP-1 gene was associated with augmented levels of macrophage infiltration [53, 54]. High expression of MCP-1 was associated with abrogation of tumorigenicity of CHO cells [53] but not of malignant mouse tumors [54]. At low tumor inocula, MCP-1 gene transfer was associated with higher tumorigenicity and lung colonizing ability, despite a lower growth of resulting lesions [54, 55]. These findings were interpreted in the light of the dual influence that TAM can exert on tumor growth [6, 50]. Expression of MCP-1/JE was detected in various rat tumors [56]. Using markers selective for monocyte-derived versus tissue macrophages, MCP-1/JE gene transfer caused recruitment of mononuclear phagocytes from the blood compartment [56]. Evidence for a role of MCP-1 in recruitment was obtained in human tumor xenografts [57].

Leukocyte infiltration in murine tumors is associated with administration of cytokines such as interferons, IL-2, or IL-4, by conventional routes or following gene transfer. Interferon, IL-12 and IL-2 induce endogenous chemokines in renal and colon cancer models [58, 59]. Thus, secondary induction of chemokines may play a pivotal role in leukocyte recruitment in tumors treated with cytokines other than chemokines.

Human tumors

Various human tumor lines express MCP-1 *in vitro* spontaneously or after exposure to inflammatory signals, and some do so *in vivo*. The latter include gliomas, histiocytomas, sarcomas and melanoma [10, 12, 60, 61]. Expression of MCP-1 was recently found in Kaposi's sarcoma (KS) *in vivo* and in KS-derived spindle cell cultures [62]. Since KS is characterized by a conspicuous macrophage infiltrate and is believed to represent a cytokine-propelled disease, production of MCP-1 may be particularly significant in this disease. Interestingly, human herpesvirus 8, likely involved in the pathogenesis of KS, encodes a constitutively active chemokine receptor which stimulates cell proliferation [63], and two chemokine-like proteins [64].

Human tumor lines of epithelial origin (breast, colon, ovary) [3, 5], release small molecular weight chemoattractant(s). For ovarian carcinoma TDCF was recently identified as MCP-1 [65].

Ovarian carcinoma is the one human tumor which has been most extensively studied for cytokine circuits between tumor cells and infiltrating leukocytes [66]. These studies have also lead to the design of therapeutic strategies targeted to TAM which gave encouraging results [67, 68]. The role of chemokines in the ping pong interaction between ovarian carcinoma cells and macrophages has been discussed [69]. Freshly isolated ovarian carcinoma cells, primary cultures, and some established cell lines were shown in early studies to release tumor-derived chemotactic factor (TDCF) activity [3–5]. These observations were recently revised [65]. Immunohistochemistry and *in situ* hybridization demonstrated that ovarian carcinoma cells and, in some tumors, also stromal elements express MCP-1. High levels of MCP-1 were measured in the ascites (but not in blood) of patients with ovarian cancer but not in the peritoneal fluid of patients with nonmalignant conditions. Production of MCP-1 and recruitment of TAM is likely to play an important role in progression of this disease because macrophage-derived cytokines promote the growth of ovarian carcinoma and its secondary implantation in peritoneal organs [70].

The expression of MCP-1 in relation to cervical cancer has been investigated by *in vitro* and *in vivo* approaches [52, 71]. Somatic cell hybrids were generated between human papillomavirus type 18 (HPV18) cells and normal cells. Only non tumorigenic hybrids expressed MCP-1, whereas it was undetectable in tumorigenic segregants and in HPV positive cervical carcinoma lines. By *in situ* hybridization, MCP-1 was detected in certain human cervical cancers. In high grade squamous intraepithelial lesions, MCP-1 expression was detected in normal, displastic and neoplastic epithelia, as well as in macrophages and endothelial cells. MCP-1 expression was most preminent at epithelial-mesenchymal function and associated with macrophage infiltration. In intraepithelial lesions, expression of MCP-1 and of the HPV oncogenes E6/E7 tended to be mutually exclusive, whereas in squamous cell carcinoma MCP-1 was expressed also in the presence of transcriptional activity of E6/E7.

Various human tumors express chemokines of the CXC family. Some neoplasms of the melanocyte lineage express GROα, and the related molecule, IL-8, which induce proliferation and migration of melanoma cells [72–74]. Transfer of the

GRO gene in an untransformed melanocytic line rendered it competent to form tumors in immunodeficient mice [72]: this effect could be related to direct growth stimulation or to promotion of an inflammatory reaction which would in turn favor tumor formation (see below). Inflammation and wound healing have in fact been implicated in initial steps of melanocyte oncogenesis [75, 76]. IL-8 is produced by various human tumor lines *in vitro*, in particular carcinomas and brain tumors, either spontaneously or after exposure to IL-1 and TNF [77, 78]. It has been speculated that IL-8 may contribute to lymphocytic infiltration in brain tumors [77]. In addition, IL-8 has angiogenic activity [79], and could thus contribute to tumor angiogenesis. A novel member of the CXC, GCP-2, was recently identified in supernatants of stimulated sarcoma cells [80]. Direct evidence that ELR+ CXC chemokines play a positive role in tumor angiogenesis has been obtained in non-small cell lung cancer [81, 82]. In this human tumor, angiogenesis appears to be regulated by a balance between pro and anti-angiogenic (IP-10) chemokines [81].

Defective systemic immunity and inflammation in cancer patients: A role for chemokines?

In terms of mounting immuno-inflammatory reactions, neoplastic disorders constitute, in a way, a paradox. As discussed above, many, if not all, tumors produce chemoattractants and are infiltrated by leukocytes: yet, it has long been known that neoplastic disorders are associated with immunosuppression and defective capacity to mount inflammatory reactions at sites other than the tumor [83]. It was repeatedly demonstrated that circulating monocytes from cancer patients have defective capacity to respond to chemoattractants [84–90]. We have speculated that tumor-derived chemokines may play a role in the two seemingly contradictory aspects of monocyte function in neoplasia (Tab. 2) [70]. Chemokines released continuously from a growing tumor, may, beyond a certain tumor size, leak into the systemic circulation. Chemoattractants are classically known to cause desensitization which, depending on the time of exposure, can be restricted to agents which use the same receptor (homologous) or involve other 7-transmembrane domain receptors. Therefore, continuous exposure to tumor-derived chemoattractants may paralyze leukocytes. A more subtle antiinflammatory action of chemoattractants depends on their effect on the receptors of the primary cytokines IL-1 and TNF [91, 92]. Chemotactic agents cause rapid shedding of the TNF receptors, most efficiently RII/p75, and of the type II IL-1 "decoy" receptor.

IL-8 was also able to induce rapid decoy RII release, though less efficiently than FMLP or C5a [91]. However, IL-8 had additive effects with other elements in the cascade of recruitment such as platelet activating factor (S. Orlando, unpublished data). Most likely, rapid shedding of the TNFR and of the IL-1 decoy R serves to

Table 2 - Chemokines as mediators of systemic anti-inflammation

Reverse gradient
Receptor desensitization
Rapid shedding of the IL-1 decoy RII
Rapid shedding of the TNFR

buffer primary proinflammatory cytokines leaking from sites of inflammation. Consistently with the concept of an anti-inflammatory potential of chemokines, systemic IL-8 inhibits local inflammatory reactions and transgenic mice overexpressing MCP-1 have impaired resistance to intracellular pathogens [93]. Thus, chemoattractant-induced continuous release of these molecules able to block IL-1 and TNF may contribute to a defective capacity to mount an inflammatory response systemically, coexisting with continuous leukocyte recruitment at the tumor site.

Monocyte functions other than chemotaxis

CC chemokines, MCP-1 in particular, affect several functions of mononuclear phagocytes related to recruitment or to effector activity. Interaction and localized digestion of extracellular matrix components is essential for phagocyte extravasation and progression in tissues. MCP-1 induces production of gelatinase and of urokinase-type plasminogen activator (uPA) [94, 95]. Concomitantly, MCP-1 augments expression of the cell surface receptor for uPA (uPA-R). Induction of gelatinase was also observed with MCP-2 and -3 [31]. Thus, CC chemokines arm monocytes with the molecular tools which allow localized and polarized digestion of extracellular matrix components during recruitment. In tumor tissues, the release of lytic enzymes by MCP-1-stimulated TAM may provide a ready-made pathway for invasion of tumor cells (counter-current invasion) and thus contribute to augmented metastasis associated with inflammation [31, 34, 50, 94, 95]. Accordingly, in one mouse model MCP-1 gene transfer augmented lung colony formation [55] and chemokines are involved in selective metastasis to the kidney in a mouse lymphoma (J.-M. Wang, unpublished data).

MCP-1 induces a respiratory burst in human monocytes, though it is a weak stimulus compared to other agonists [12, 96]. Natural MCP-1 was reported to induce IL-1 and IL-6 but not TNF production [96]. In another study recombinant MCP-1 had little effect on IL-6 release (M. Sironi, unpublished data). Human MCP-1 induced monocyte cytostasis for a tumor line [12] or synergized with bacterial products (but not with interferonγ, (IFNγ)) in stimulation of mouse macrophage cytotoxicity [97, 98]. In an interesting and intriguing recent study, human MCP-1 inhibited induction of the NO synthase in the macrophage cell line J774 [99]. TAM have reduced NO synthase activity [100]. If confirmed, this finding would suggest that MCP-1 could account for both recruitment and concomitant partial functional deactivation of TAM (see below).

Therapeutic potential of chemokines: Antiangiogenesis

In general, the spectrum of action of chemokines tends to be restricted to leukocytes, but recent evidence suggests that some members of this superfamily of inflammatory mediators may affect EC function. IL-8, GROα and other CXC chemokines were reported to induce EC migration and proliferation *in vitro* and to be angiogenic *in vivo* [79]. The expression of high affinity receptors and responsiveness to IL-8 of EC has however been the object of conflicting results [101, 102].

In common with platelet factor 4, IP10 was shown to have angiostatic properties *in vivo* and represent the ultimate mediator of the anti-angiogenic activity of IL-12 [103], though conflicting results have been obtained as to its capacity to inhibit bFGF-induced proliferation of HUVEC *in vitro* [104, 105]. A three amino acid motif (ELR), is conserved in members of the CXC family which activate neutrophils. Recent results, including the action of molecules with or without the ELR motif and the activity of IL-8 muteins, suggest that the presence or absence of an ELR motif dictates whether CXC chemokines induce or inhibit angiogenesis [106]. However, the observation that GROβ inhibits angiogenesis is not consistent with this model of function [107].

Three types of chemokine binding sites have been identified. The presence and type of signaling chemokine receptors on EC is controversial [79, 101, 102]. The promiscuous chemokine receptor identical to the Duffy blood group antigen (DARC) is expressed by EC at post-capillary venules *in vivo*, but not by endothelial cells *in vitro* [108]. Finally, heparin and heparin-like proteoglycans on endothelial cells present at least some chemokines to leukocytes in the multistep process of recruitment [109].

Thus, certain chemokines, such as IP-10 have anti-angiogenic activity, and represent the ultimate mediator in the anti-tumor action of a cytokine cascade involving IL-12 and IFNγ. After gene transfer in certain tumors, other cellular targets (e.g. T cells) may play a role in the antitumor activity of IP-10.

Therapeutic potential of chemokines: Attraction of dendritic cells

Cytokine gene transfer into tumor cells has resulted in tumor rejection in experimental systems and is undergoing evaluation in human tumors. The antitumor activity of cytokine gene transfer is associated with distinct patterns of leukocyte infiltration (for review see [110]). Although it is likely that chemokines play a pivotal role in determining the timing, type and amount of infiltrate under these conditions, detailed analysis is at present lacking.

Chemokines have been used in gene transfer studies. Depending on the tumor type, MCP-1 gene transfer has been associated with abrogation of tumorigenicity, reduced growth rate, augmented tumor takes or metastasis or no effect [52, 54, 55, 111, 112]. Antitumor activity and activation of specific immunity has been observed after gene transfer of IP-10, TCA3, RANTES, lymphotactin and MCP-3 [110, 113–116], see also below.

A major goal of immunotherapeutic approaches to neoplasia is activation of specific anti-tumor immunity. In this perspective, dendritic cells may be a crucial determinant of success or failure. Recent results suggest that dendritic cells (DC) express receptors for and respond to chemokines [22, 117, 118].

DC precursors originate in the bone marrow and subsequently migrate into peripheral tissues and primary lymphoid organs, where they efficiently take up and process soluble antigens. After capture of antigen in tissues, DC migrate via the afferent lymphatics to draining lymphnodes or via blood to spleen, where they stimulate T cells [119]. As the molecules controlling these events are unknown, we investigated which chemotactic factors could attract this cell population and regulate their trafficking in tissues [117].

For these experiments, DC were obtained from peripheral blood precursor cells cultured in the presence of GM-CSF and IL-4 or IL-13 [120, 121]. These cells were CD1a$^+$, MHC class II^{++}, CD14$^-$, CD3$^-$ and CD20$^-$ and behaved as classical immature DC being active in eliciting the proliferation of naïve T lymphocytes and showing a strong ability to take up FITC-dextran [121]. In a classical microwell chemotaxis assay these cells migrated in response to a selected pattern of CC chemokines, such as MCP-3, RANTES and MIP1α and to two prototypic chemotactic factors, fMLP and C5a [117] (Tab. 3). MCP-1 and MCP-2, two other CC chemokines and all of the CXC chemokines tested (IL-8, IP-10 and GROβ) were inactive. Peak active concentrations and the percentage of input cells migrating in response to CC chemokines were comparable to those observed with monocytes.

MCP-3, MIP-1α and RANTES showed a complex pattern of cross-desensitization suggesting the presence of multiple promiscuous receptors on these cells. In northern blot studies it was found that DC express the CCR1, CCR2, CCR5 as well as CXCR2 and CXCR4 receptors. DC respond to SDF1 but not to IL-8 and MCP-1 *in vitro* in spite of expression of CCR2 and CXCR2 mRNA [118].

Transgenic mice for MCP-1, in which MCP-1 is constitutively expressed in the epidermis under the control of human keratin 14 promoter, respond to a contact hypersensitivity challenge with an increased lichenoid infiltration of monocytes, T lymphocytes and CD45$^+$, I-A$^+$ cells that assumed a dendritic morphology *in situ* [122]. We speculate that MCP-1 may attract monocytes to the skin, where these cells find an environment (e.g. GM-CSF) conducible to DC differentiation.

Table 3 - Chemoattractant activity on dendritic cells

Family	Active	Inactive
CXC	SDF-1	IL-8, GROß, IP-10
CC	MCP-3, MCP-4, MIP-1α	MCP-1, MCP-2
	MIP-1β, MIP-5	Eotaxin
	RANTES, MIP-3α*, MDC	
C	–	lymphotactin
Classical, peptides	C5a, FMLP	–
Classical, lipids	PAF	–

*Active on CD34-derived DC but not on monocyte-derived DC.

Macrophage derived chemokine (MDC) is a recently identified CC chemokine, which, unlike related molecules, is located on chromosome 16 and has a rather distant relationship with other family members [22]. We recently found that MDC has an ED50 100 fold lower for activated NK cells and DC than for monocytes [22]. Moreover, it is expressed by DC in addition to macrophages. We speculate that molecules such as SDF-1 and MDC may contribute to directing the "normal" trafficking of DC in the absence of antigen or inflammation, whereas inducible chemokines may underlie the dramatic changes in route and trafficking after exposure to antigenic or inflammatory stimulation.

Recently, for the first time, a chemokine selectively active on monocyte derived versus CD34+ cell-derived DC was identified [123]. The molecule known as MIP-3α/LARC/exodus was found to selectively attract CD34 derived DC and not monocyte-derived DC. MIP-3α/LARC/exodus interacts with CCR6 and its differential action on DC populations reflects differential receptor expression.

In the context of our interest in chemokines and DC, we recently transfected tumor cells with MCP-3 (A. Vecchi et al., unpublished data). After MCP-3 gene transfer, P815 mastocytoma cells grew and underwent rejection. MCP-3-elicited rejection was associated with resistance to subsequent challenge with parental cells. MCP-3 elicited rejection was associated with profound alterations of leukocyte infiltration. TAM already present in copious number, T cells, eosinophils and neutrophils increased in tumor tissues after MCP-3 gene transfer. DC (e.g. Dec205+, high MHC class II+ cells) did not increase substantially in the tumor mass. However, in peritumoral tissues, DC accumulated in perivascular areas. MCP-3-transfected tumor cells grew normally in nude mice. Increased accumulation of macrophages and PMN was evident also in nude mice. Antibodies against CD4, CD8 and IFNγ, but not against IL-4, inhibited rejection of MCP-3 transfected P815 cells. An anti-

PMN mAb caused only a retardation of MCP-3 elicited tumor rejection. Thus, MCP-3 gene transfer elicits tumor rejection by activating type I T cell-dependent immunity. It is tempting to speculate that altered trafficking of antigen presenting cells, which express receptors and respond to MCP-3, together with recruitment of activated T cells, underlies activation of specific immunity by MCP-3 transfected cells.

Concluding remarks

Chemokines play a dual role in the regulation of tumor growth and metastasis. Certain chemokines are produced by tumor cells and, by attracting macrophages and endothelial cells, provide optimal conditions for tumor growth and progression. We also speculate that chemokines leaking from sites of tumor growth may contribute to systemic impairment of the capacity to mount immune and inflammatory reactions frequently observed in advanced neoplasia. Conversely, the anti-angiogenic activity of chemokines and their capacity to recruit and activate immunocompetent cells can be exploited therapeutically in gene transfer studies.

A better understanding of the physiological role of chemokines in directing the traffic of dendritic cells and NK cells, crucial for the activation and orientation of specific immunity, may provide a basis for less empirical design of chemokine-based therapeutic strategies.

References

1   Ward PA, Remold HG, David JR (1970) The production by antigen-stimulated lymphocytes of a lekotactic factor distinct from migration inhibitory factor. *Cell Immunol* 1: 162–174

2   Meltzer MS, Stevenson MM, Leonard EJ (1977) Characterization of macrophage chemotaxis in tumor cell cultures and comparison with lymphocyte-derived chemotactic factors. *Cancer Res* 37: 721–725

3   Bottazzi B, Polentarutti N, Acero R, Balsari A, Boraschi D, Ghezzi P, Salmona M, Mantovani A (1983) Regulation of the macrophage content of neoplasms by chemoattractants. *Science* 220: 210–212

4   Bottazzi B, Polentarutti N, Balsari A, Boraschi D, Ghezzi P, Salmona M, Mantovani A (1983) Chemotactic activity for mononuclear phagocytes of culture supernatants from murine and human tumor cells: evidence for a role in the regulation of the macrophage content of neoplastic tissues. *Int J Cancer* 31: 55–63

5   Bottazzi B, Ghezzi P, Taraboletti G, Salmona M, Colombo N, Bonazzi C, Mangioni C, Mantovani A (1985) Tumor-derived chemotactic factor(s) from human ovarian carcinoma: evidence for a role in the regulation of macrophage content of neoplastic tissues. *Int J Cancer* 36: 167–173

6   Mantovani A, Bottazzi B, Colotta F, Sozzani S, Ruco L (1992) The origin and function of tumor-associated macrophages. *Immunol Today* 13: 265–270

7   Valente AJ, Fowler SR, Sprague EA, Kelley JL, Suenram CA, Schwartz CJ (1984) Initial characterization of a peripheral blood mononuclear cell chemoattractant derived from cultured arterial smooth muscle cells. *Am J Pathol* 117: 409–417

8   Zullo JN, Cochran BH, Huang AS, Stiles CD (1985) Platelet-derived growth factor and double-stranded ribonucleic acids stimulate expression of the same genes in 3T3 cells. *Cell* 43: 793–800

9   Rollins BJ, Morrison ED, Stiles CD (1988) Cloning and expression of JE, a gene inducible by platelet-derived growth factor and whose product has cytokine-like properties. *Proc Natl Acad Sci USA* 85: 3738–3742

10 Yoshimura T, Robinson EA, Tanaka S, Appella E, Kuratsu J, Leonard EJ (1989) Purification and amino acid analysis of two human glioma-derived monocyte chemoattractants. *J Exp Med* 169: 1449–1459

11 Matsushima K, Larsen CG, DuBois GC, Oppenheim JJ (1989) Purification and characterization of a novel monocyte chemotactic and activating factor produced by a human myelomonocytic cell line. *J Exp Med* 169: 1485–1490

12 Zachariae CO, Anderson AO, Thompson HL, Appella E, Mantovani A, Oppenheim JJ, Matsushima K (1990) Properties of monocyte chemotactic and activating factor (MCAF) purified from a human fibrosarcoma cell line. *J Exp Med* 171: 2177–2182

13 Van Damme J, Decock B, Lenaerts JP, Conings R, Bertini R, Mantovani A, Billiau A (1989) Identification by sequence analysis of chemotactic factors for monocytes produced by normal and transformed cells stimulated with virus, double-stranded RNA or cytokine. *Eur J Immunol* 19: 2367–2373

14 Graves DT, Jiang YL, Williamson MJ, Valente AJ (1989) Identifcation of monocyte chemotactic activity produced by malignant cells. *Science* 245: 1490–1493

15 Furutani Y, Nomura H, Notake M, Oyamada Y, Fukuy T, Yamada M, Larsen CG, Oppenheim JJ, Matsushima K (1989) Cloning and sequencing of the cDNA for human monocyte chemotactic and activating factor (MCAF). *Biochem Biophys Res Commun* 159: 248–255

16 Yoshimura T, Yuhki N, Moore SK, Appella E, Lerman MI, Leonard EJ (1989) Human monocyte chemoattractant proein-1 (MCP-1). Full-length cDNA cloning, expression in mitogen-stimulation blood mononuclear meukocytes, and sequence similarity to mouse competence gene JE. *FEBS Lett* 244: 487–493

17 Bottazzi B, Colotta F, Sica A, Nobili N, Mantovani A (1990) A chemoattractant expressed in human sarcoma cells (tumor-derived chemotactic factor, TDCF) is identical to monocyte chemoattractant protein-1/monocyte chemotactic and activating factor (MCP-1/MCAF). *Int J Cancer* 45: 795–797

18 Baggiolini M, Dewald B, Moser B (1997) Human chemokines: An update. *Annu Rev Immunol* 15: 675–705

19 Feldmann M, Brennan FM, Maini RN (1996) Rheumatoid arthritis. *Cell* 85: 307–310

20 Hieshima K, Imai T, Opdenakker G, Vandamme J, Kusuda J, Tei H, Sakaki Y, Takatsu-

ki K, Miura R, Yoshie O, Nomiyama H (1997) Molecular cloning of a novel human CC chemokine liver and activation-regulated chemokine (LARC) expressed in liver – Chemotactic activity for lymphocytes and gene localization on chromosome. *J Biol Chem* Vol. 272, Iss. 9: 5846–5853

21 Imai T, Yoshida T, Baba M, Nishimura M, Kakizaki M, Yoshie O (1996) Molecular cloning of a novel T cell-directed CC chemokine expressed in thymus by signal sequence trap using Epstein-Barr virus vector. *J Biol Chem* 271: 21514–21521

22 Godiska R, Chantry D, Raport CJ, Sozzani S, Allavena P, Leviten D, Mantovani A, Gray PW (1997) Human macrophage derived chemokine (MDC) a novel chemoattractant for monocytes, monocyte derived dendritic cells, and natural killer cells. *J Exp Med* 185: 1595–1604

23 Catterall JB, Gardner MJ, Jones LMH, Thompson GA, Turner GA (1994) A precise, rapid and sensitive *in vitro* assay to measure the adhesion of ovarian tumour cells to peritoneal mesothelial cells. *Cancer Lett* 87: 199–203

24 Robinson EA, Yoshimura T, Leonard EJ, Tanaka S, Griffin PR, Shabanowitz J, Hunt DF, Appella E (1989) Complete amino acid sequence of a human monocyte chemoattrac-tant, a putative mediator of cellular immune reactions. *Proc Natl Acad Sci USA* 86: 1850–1854

25 Decock B, Conings R, Lenaerts JP, Billiau A, Van Damme J (1990) Identification of the monocyte chemotactic protein from human osteosarcoma cells and monocytes: detection of a novel N-terminally processed form. *Biochem Biophys Res Commun* 167: 904– 909

26 Woldemar Carr M, Roth SJ, Luther E, Rose SS, Springer TA (1994) Monocyte chemoat-tractant protein-1 acts as a T-lymphocyte chemoattractant. *Proc Natl Acad Sci USA* 91: 3652–3656

27 Jiang Y, Valente AJ, Williamson MJ, Zhang L, Graves DT (1990) Post-translational modification of a monocyte-specific chemoattractant synthesized by glioma, osteosar-coma, and vascular smooth muscle cells. *J Biol Chem* 265: 18318–18321

28 Gronenborn AM, Clore GM (1991) Modeling the three-dimensional structure of the monocyte chemo-attractant and activating protein MCAF/MCP-1 on the basis of the solution structure of interleukin-8. *Protein Eng* 4: 263–269

29 Lodi PJ, Garrett DS, Kuszewski J, Tsang MLS, Weatherbee JA, Leonard WJ, Gronen-born AM, Clore GM (1994) High-resolution solution structure of the beta chemokine Hmip-1 beta by multidimensional NMR. *Science* 263: 1762–1767

30 Paolini JF, Willard D, Consler T, Luther M, Krangel MS (1994) The chemokines IL-8, monocyte chemoattractant protein-1, and I-309 are monomers at physiologically rele-vant concentrations. *J Immunol* 153: 2704–2717

31 Van Damme J, Proost P, Lenaerts JP, Opdenakker G (1992) Structural and functional identification of two human, tumor-derived monocyte chemotactic proteins (MCP-2 and MCP-3) belonging to the chemokine family. *J Exp Med* 176: 59–65

32 Proost P, Vanleuven P, Wuyts A, Ebberink R, Opdenakker G, Van Damme J (1995) Chemical synthesis, purification and folding of the human monocyte chemotactic pro-teins MCP-2 and MCP-3 into biologically active chemokines. *Cytokine* 7: 97–104

33   Minty A, Chalon P, Guillemot JC, Kaghad M, Liauzun P, Magazin M, Miloux B, Minty C, Ramond P, Vita N, Lupker J, Shire D, Ferrara P, Caput D (1993) Molecular cloning of the MCP-3 chemokine gene and regulation of its expression. *Eur Cytokine Netw* 4: 99–110

34   Opdenakker G, Froyen G, Fiten P, Proost P, Van Damme J (1993) Human monocyte chemotactic protein-3 (MCP-3): molecular cloning of the cDNA and comparison with other chemokines. *Biochem Biophys Res Commun* 191: 535–542

35   Opdenakker G, Fiten P, Nys G, Froyen G, Vanroy N, Speleman F, Laureys G, Van Damme J (1994) The human MCP-3 gene (SCYA7): Cloning, sequence analysis, and assignment to the CC chemokine gene cluster on chromosome 17q11.2-q12. *Genomics* 21: 403–408

36   Mehrabian M, Sparkes RS, Mohandas T, Fogelman AM, Lusis AJ (1991) Localization of monocyte chemotactic protein-1 gene (SCYA2) to human chromosome 17q11.2-q21.1. *Genomics* 9: 200–203

37   Rollins BJ, Morton CC, Ledbetter DH, Eddy RLJ, Shows TB (1991) Assignment of the human small inducible cytokine A2 gene, SCYA2 (encoding JE or MCP-1), to 17q11.2-12: evolutionary relatedness of cytokines clustered at the same locus. *Genomics* 10: 489–492

38   VanCoillie E, Fiten P, Nomiyama H, Sakaki Y, Miura R, Yoshie O, Van Damme J, Opdenakker G (1997) The human MCP-2 gene (SCYA8): Cloning, sequence analysis, tissue expression, and assignment to the CC chemokine gene contig on chromosome 17q11.2. *Genomics* Vol 40, Iss 2: 323–331

39   Chang HC, Hsu F, Freeman GJ, Griffin JD, Reinherz EL (1989) Cloning and expression of a gamma-interferon-inducible gene in monocytes: a new member of a cytokine gene family. *Int Immunol* 1: 388–397

40   Shyy YJ, Li YS, Kolattukudy PE (1990) Structure of human monocyte chemotactic protein gene and its regulation by TPA. *Biochem Biophys Res Commun* 169: 346–351

41   Ueda A, Okuda K, Ohno S, Shirai A, Igarashi T, Matsunaga K, Fukushima J, Kawamoto S, Ishigatsubo Y, Okubo T (1994) NF-kappa B and Sp1 regulate transcription of the human monocyte chemoattractant protein-1 gene. *J Immunol* 153: 2052–2063

42   Colotta F, Borre A, Wang JM, Tattanelli M, Maddalena F, Polentarutti N, Peri G, Mantovani A (1992) Expression of a monocyte chemotactic cytokine by human mononuclear phagocytes. *J Immunol* 148: 760–765

43   Rollins BJ, Stier P, Ernst T, Wong GG (1989) The human homolog of the JE gene encodes a monocyte secretory protein. *Mol Cell Biol* 9: 4687–4695

44   Van Damme J, Decock B, Bertini R, Conings R, Lenaerts JP, Put W, Opdenakker G, Mantovani A (1991) Production and identification of natural monocyte chemotactic protein from virally infected murine fibroblasts. Relationship with the product of the mouse competence (JE) gene. *Eur J Biochem* 199: 223–229

45   Thirion S, Nys G, Fiten P, Masure S, Van Damme J, Opdenakker G (1994) Mouse macrophage derived monocyte chemotactic protein-3: cDNA cloning and identification as MARC/FIC. *Biochem Biophys Res Commun* 201: 493–499

46   Kulmburg PA, Huber NE, Scheer BJ, Wrann M, Baumruker T (1992) Immunoglobulin E plus antigen challenge induces a novel intercrine/chemokine in mouse mast cells. *J Exp Med* 176: 1773–1778

47   Heinrich JN, Ryseck RP, Macdonald-Bravo H, Bravo R (1993) The product of a novel growth factor-activated gene, fic, is a biologically active CC-type cytokine. *Mol Cell Biol* 13: 2020–2030

48   Bucana CD, Fabra A, Sanchez R, Fidler IJ (1992) Different patterns of macrophage infiltration into allogeneic-murine and xenogeneic-human neoplasms growing in nude mice. *Am J Pathol* 141: 1225–1236

49   Heuff G, van der Ende MB, Boutkan H, Prevoo W, Bayon LG, Fleuren GJ, Beelen RH, Meijer S, Dijkstra CD (1993) Macrophage populations in different stages of induced hepatic metastases in rats: an immunohistochemical analysis. *Scand J Immunol* 38: 10–16

50   Opdenakker G, Van Damme J (1992) Chemotactic factors, passive invasion and metastasis of cancer cells. *Immunol Today* 13: 463–464

51   Walter S, Bottazzi B, Govoni D, Colotta F, Mantovani A (1991) Macrophage infiltration and growth of sarcoma clones expressing different amounts of monocyte chemotactic protein/JE. *Int J Cancer* 49: 431–435

52   Hirose K, Hakozaki M, Nyunoya Y, Kobayashi Y, Matsushita K, Takenouchi T, Mikata A, Mukaida N, Matsushima K (1995) Chemokine gene transfection into tumour cells reduced tumorigenicity in nude mice in association with neutrophilic infiltration. *Br J Cancer* 72: 708–714

53   Rollins BJ, Sunday ME (1991) Suppression of tumor formation *in vivo* by expression of the JE gene in malignant cells. *Mol Cell Biol* 11: 3125–3131

54   Bottazzi B, Walter S, Govoni D, Colotta F, Mantovani A (1992) Monocyte chemotactic cytokine gene transfer modulates macrophage infiltration, growth, and susceptibility to IL-2 therapy of a murine melanoma. *J Immunol* 148: 1280–1285

55   Mantovani A, Bottazzi B, Sozzani S, Peri G, Allavena P, Dong QG, Vecchi A, Colotta F (1993) Cytokine regulation of tumour-associated macrophages. *Res Immunol* 144: 280–283

56   Yamashiro S, Takeya M, Nishi T, Kuratsu J, Yoshimura T, Ushio Y, Takahashi K (1994) Tumor-derived monocyte chemoattractant protein-1 induces intratumoral infiltration of monocyte-derived macrophage subpopulation in transplanted rat tumors. *Am J Pathol* 145: 856–867

57   Melani C, Pupa SM, Stoppacciaro A, Menard S, Colnaghi MI, Parmiani G, Colombo MP (1995) An *in vivo* model to compare human leukocyte infiltration in carcinoma xenografts producing different chemokines. *Int J Cancer* 62: 572–578

58   Sonouchi K, Hamilton TA, Tannenbaum CS, Tubbs RR, Bukowski R, Finke JH (1994) Chemokine gene expression in the murine renal cell carcinoma, renca, following treatment *in vivo* with Interferon-alpha and Interleukin-2. *Am J Pathol* 144: 747–755

59   Tannenbaum CS, Wicker N, Armstrong D, Tubbs R, Finke J, Bukowski RM, Hamilton TA (1996) Cytokine and chemokine expression in tumors of mice receiving systemic therapy with IL-12. *J Immunol* 156: 693–699

60 Graves DT, Barnhill R, Galanopoulos T, Antoniades HN. Expression of monocyte chemotactic protein-1 in human melanoma *in vivo*. *Am J Pathol* 1992 140: 9–14

61 Takeya M, Yoshimura T, Leonard EJ, Kato T, Okabe H, Takahashi K (1991) Production of monocyte chemoattractant protein-1 by malignant fibrous histiocytoma: relation to the origin of histiocyte-like cells. *Exp Mol Pathol* 54: 61–71

62 Sciacca FL, Stürzl M, Bussolino F, Sironi M, Brandstetter H, Zietz C, Zhou D, Matteucci C, Peri G, Sozzani S, Benelli R, Arese M, Albini A, Colotta F, Mantovani A (1994) Expression of adhesion molecules, platelet-activating factor, and chemokines by Kaposi's sarcoma cells. *J Immunol* 153: 4816–4825

63 Arvanitakis L, Geras-Raaka E, Varma A, Gershergorn MC, Cesarman E (1997) Human herpesvirus KSHV encodes a constitutively active G-protein-coupled receptor linked to cell proliferation. *Nature* 385: 347–350

64 Moore PS, Boshoff C, Weiss RA, Chang Y (1996) Molecular mimicry of human cytokine and cytokine response pathway genes by KSHV. *Science* 274: 1739–1744

65 Negus RP, Stamp GW, Relf MG, Burke F, Malik ST, Bernasconi S, Allavena P, Sozzani S, Mantovani A, Balkwill FR (1995) The detection and localization of monocyte chemoattractant protein-1 (MCP-1) in human ovarian cancer. *J Clin Invest* 95: 2391–2396

66 Burke F, Relf M, Negus R, Balkwill F (1996) A cytokine profile of normal and malignant ovary. *Cytokine* 8: 578–585

67 Allavena P, Peccatori F, Maggioni D, Erroi A, Sironi M, Colombo N, Lissoni A, Galazka A, Meiers W, Mangioni C, Mantovani A (1990) Intraperitoneal recombinant gamma-interferon in patients with recurrent ascitic ovarian carcinoma: modulation of cytotoxicity and cytokine production in tumor-associated effectors and of major histocompatibility antigen expression on tumor cells. *Cancer Res* 50: 7318–7323

68 Colombo N, Peccatori F, Paganin C, Bini S, Brandely M, Mangioni C, Mantovani A, Allavena P (1992) Anti-tumor and immunomodulatory activity of intraperitoneal IFN-gamma in ovarian carcinoma patients with minimal residual tumor after chemotherapy. *Int J Cancer* 51: 42–46

69 Evans R (1972) Macrophages in syngeneic animal tumours. *Transplantation* 14: 468–470

70 Mantovani A (1994) Tumor-associated macrophages in neoplastic progression: A paradigm for the *in vivo* function of chemokines. *Lab Invest* 71: 5–16

71 Riethdorf L, Riethdorf S, Gutzlaff K, Prall F, Loning T (1996) Differential expression of the monocyte chemoattractant protein-1 gene in human papillomavirus-16-infected squamous intraepithelial lesions and squamous cell carcinomas of the cervix uteri. *Am J Pathol* 149: 1469–1476

72 Balentien E, Mufson BE, Shattuck RL, Derynck R, Richmond A (1991) Effects of MGSA/GRO alpha on melanocyte transformation. *Oncogene* 6: 1115–1124

73 Wang JM, Taraboletti G, Matsushima K, Van Damme J, Mantovani A (1990) Induction of haptotactic migration of melanoma cells by neutrophil activating protein/interleukin-8 *Biochem Biophys Res Commun* 169: 165–170

74 Schadendorf D, Moller A, Algermissen B, Worm M, Sticherling M, Czarnetzki BM

(1993) IL-8 produced by human malignant melanoma cells *in vitro* is an essential autocrine growth factor. *J Immunol* 151: 2667–2675

75 Mintz B, Silvers WK (1993) Transgenic mouse model of malignant skin melanoma. *Proc Natl Acad Sci USA* 90: 8817–8821

76 Medrano EE, Farooqui JZ, Boissy RE, Boissy YL, Akadiri B, Nordlund JJ (1993) Chronic growth stimulation of human adult melanocytes by inflammatory mediators *in vitro*: implications for nevus formation and initial steps in melanocyte oncogenesis. *Proc Natl Acad Sci USA* 90: 1790–1794

77 Van Meir E, Ceska M, Effenberger F, Walz A, Grouzmann E, Desbaillets I, Frei K, Fontana A, de Tribolet N (1992) Interleukin-8 is produced in neoplastic and infectious diseases of the human central nervous system. *Cancer Res* 52: 4297–4305

78 Sakamoto K, Masuda T, Mita S, Ishiko T, Nakashima Y, Arakawa H, Egami H, Harada S, Matsushima K, Ogawa M (1992) Interleukin-8 is constitutively and commonly produced by various human carcinoma cell lines. *Int J Clin Lab Res* 22: 216–219

79 Koch AE, Polverini PJ, Kunkel SL, Harlow LA, DiPietro LA, Elner VM, Elner SG, Strieter RM (1992) Interleukin-8 as a macrophage-derived mediator of angiogenesis. *Science* 258: 1798–1801

80 Proost P, De Wolf Peeters C, Conings R, Opdenakker G, Billiau A, Van Damme J (1993) Identification of a novel granulocyte chemotactic protein (GCP-2) from human tumor cells. *In vitro* and *in vivo* comparison with natural forms of GRO, IP-10, and IL-8. *J Immunol* 150: 1000–1010

81 Arenberg DA, Kunkel SL, Polverini PJ, Morris SB, Burdick MD, Glass MC, Taub DT, Iannettoni MD, Whyte TI, Strieter RM (1996) Interferon-gamma-inducible protein 10 (IP-10) is an angiostatic factor that inhibits human non-small cell lung cancer (NSCLC) tumorigenesis and spontaneous metastases. *J Exp Med* 184: 981–992

82 Smith DR, Polverini PJ, Kunkel SL, Orringer MB, Whyte RI, Burdick MD, Wilke CA, Strieter RM (1994) Inhibition of IL-8 attenuates angiogenesis in bronchogenic carcinoma. *J Exp Med* 179: 1409–1415

83 Snyderman R, Cianciolo GJ (1984) Immunosuppressive activity of the retroviral envelope protein P15E and its possible relationship to neoplasia. Immunol Today 5: 240–244

84 Boechter D, Leonard EJ. Abnormal monocyte chemotactic response in mice. *J Natl Cancer Inst* 1974 52: 1091–1099

85 Normann SJ, Schardt M, Sorkin E (1981) Biphasic depression of macrophage function after tumor transplantation. *Int J Cancer* 28: 185–190

86 Normann SJ, Sorkin E (1976) Cell-specific defect in monocyte function during tumor growth. *J Natl Cancer Inst* 57: 135–140

87 Normann SJ, Sorkin E (1977) Inhibition of macrophage chemotaxis by neoplastic and other rapidly proliferating cells *in vitro*. *Cancer Res* 37: 705–711

88 Stevenson MM, Meltzer MS (1976) Depressed chemotactic responses *in vitro* of peritoneal macrophages from tumor-bearing mice. *J Natl Cancer Inst* 57: 847–852

89 Snyderman R, Pike MC (1976) An inhibitor of macrophage chemotaxis produced by neoplasms. *Science* 192: 370–372

90 Cianciolo GJ, Hunter J, Silva J, Haskill JS, Snyderman R (1981) Inhibitors of monocyte responses to chemotaxins are present in human cancerous effusions and react with monoclonal antibodies to the P15(E) structural protein of retroviruses. *J Clin Invest* 68: 831–844

91 Colotta F, Orlando S, Fadlon EJ, Sozzani S, Matteucci C, Mantovani A (1995) Chemoattractants induce rapid release of the interleukin 1 type II decoy receptor in human polymorphonuclear cells. *J Exp Med* 181: 2181–2188

92 Porteu F, Nathan C (1990) Shedding of tumor necrosis factor receptor by activated human neutrophils. *J Exp Med* 172: 599–607

93 Rutledge BJ, Rayburn H, Rosenberg R, North RJ, Gladue RP, Corless CL, Rollins BJ (1995) High level monocyte chemoattractant protein-1 expression in transgenic mice increases their susceptibility to intracellular pathogens. *J Immunol* 155: 4838–4843

94 Opdenakker G, Van Damme J (1992) Cytokines and proteases in invasive processes: molecular similarities between inflammation and cancer. *Cytokine* 4: 251–258

95 Mantovani A, Sozzani S, Bottazzi B, Peri G, Sciacca FL, Locati M, Colotta F (1993) Monocyte chemotactic protein-1 (MCP-1): signal transduction and involvement in the regulation of macrophage traffic in normal and neoplastic tissues. *Adv Exp Med Biol* 351: 47–54

96 Jiang Y, Beller DI, Frendl G, Graves DT (1992) Monocyte chemoattractant protein-1 regulates adhesion molecule expression and cytokine production in human monocytes. *J Immunol* 148: 2423–2428

97 Singh RK, Berry K, Matsushima K, Yasumoto K, Fidler IJ (1993) Synergism between human monocyte chemotactic and activating factor and bacterial products for activation of tumoricidal properties in murine macrophages. *J Immunol* 151: 2786–2793

98 Asano T, An T, Jia SF, Kleinerman ES (1996) Altered monocyte chemotactic and activating factor gene expression in human glioblastoma cell lines increased their susceptibility to cytotoxicity. *J Leukocyte Biol* 59: 916–924

99 Rojas A, Delgado R, Glaria L, Palacios M (1993) Monocyte chemotactic protein-1 inhibits the induction of nitric oxide synthase in J774 cells. *Biochem Biophys Res Commun* 196: 274–279

100 DiNapoli MR, Calderon CL, Lopez DM (1996) The altered tumoricidal capacity of macrophages isolated from tumor-bearing mice is related to reduced expression of the inducible nitric oxide synthase gene. *J Exp Med* 183: 1323–1329

101 Schonbeck U, Brandt E, Petersen F, Flad HD, Loppnow H (1995) IL-8 specifically binds to endothelial but not to smooth muscle cells. *J Immunol* 154: 2375–2383

102 Petzelbauer P, Watson CA, Pfau SE, Pober JS (1995) IL-8 and angiogenesis: Evidence that human endothelial cells lack receptors and do not respond to IL-8 *in vitro*. *Cytokine* 7: 267–272

103 Voest EE, Kenyon BM, O'Reilly MS, Truitt G, D'Amato RJ, Folkman J (1995) Inhibition of angiogenesis *in vivo* by interleukin-12. *J Natl Cancer Inst* 87: 581–586

104 Luster AD, Greenberg SM, Leder P (1995) The IP-10 chemokine binds to a specific cell

surface heparan sulfate site shared with platelet factor 4 and inhibits endothelial cell proliferation. *J Exp Med* 182: 219–231

105 Angiolillo AL, Sgadari C, Taub DD, Liao F, Farber JM, Maheshwari S, Kleinman HK, Reaman GH, Tosato G (1995) Human interferon-inducible protein 10 is a potent inhibitor of angiogenesis *in vivo*. *J Exp Med* 182: 155–162

106 Strieter RM, Polverini PJ, Kunkel SL, Arenberg DA, Burdick MD, Kasper J, Dzuiba J, Van Damme J, Walz A, Marriott D, Chan SY, Roczniak S, Shanafelt AB (1995) The functional role of the ELR motif in CXC chemokine-mediated angiogenesis . *J Biol Chem* 270: 27348–27357

107 Cao YH, Chen C, Weatherbee JA, Tsang M, Folkman J (1995) GRO-beta, a -CXC-chemokine, is an angiogenesis inhibitor that suppresses the growth of Lewis lung carcinoma in mice. *J Exp Med* 182: 2069–2077

108 Peiper SC, Wang ZX, Neote K, Martin AW, Showell HJ, Conklyn MJ, Ogborne K, Hadley TJ, Lu ZH, Hesselgesser J, Horuk R (1995) The Duffy antigen receptor for chemokines (DARC) is expressed in endothelial cells of Duffy negative individuals who lack the erythrocyte receptor. *J Exp Med* 181: 1311–1317

109 Rot A (1992) Endothelial cell binding of NAP-1/IL-8: role in neutrophil emigration. *Immunol Today* 13: 291–294

110 Musiani P, Modesti A, Giovarelli M, Cavallo F, Colombo MP, Lollini PL, Forni G (1997) Cytokines, tumor-cell death and immunogenicity: a question of choice. *Immunol Today* 18: 32–36

111 Clauss M, Gerlach M, Gerlach H, Brett J, Wang F, Familletti PC, Pan YC, Olander JV, Connolly DT, Stern D (1990) Vascular permeability factor: a tumor-derived polypeptide that induces endothelial cell and monocyte procoagulant activity, and promotes monocyte migration. *J Exp Med* 172: 1535–1545

112 Pardoll DM (1995) Paracrine cytokine adjuvants in cancer immunotherapy. *Annu Rev Immunol* 13: 399–415

113 Luster AD, Leder P (1993) IP-10, a -CXC- chemokine, elicits a potent thymus-dependent antitumor response *in vivo*. *J Exp Med* 178: 1057–1065

114 Laning J, Kawasaki H, Tanaka E, Luo Y, Dorf ME (1994) Inhibition of *in vivo* tumor growth by the beta chemokine, TCA3. *J Immunol* 153: 4625–4635

115 Mulé JJ, Custer M, Averbook B, Yang JC, Weber JS, Goeddel DV, Rosenberg SA, Schall TJ (1996) RANTES secretion by gene-modified tumor cells results in loss of tumorigenicity *in vivo*: role of immune cell subpopulations. *Hum Gene Ther* 7: 1545–1553

116 Dilloo D, Bacon K, Holden W, Zhong WY, Burdach S, Zlotnik A, Brenner M (1996) Combined chemokine and cytokine gene transfer enhances antitumor immunity. *Nature Med* 2: 1090–1095

117 Sozzani S, Sallusto F, Luini W, Zhou D, Piemonti L, Allavena P, Van Damme J, Valitutti S, Lanzavecchia A, Mantovani A (1995) Migration of dendritic cells in response to formyl peptides, C5a and a distinct set of chemokines. *J Immunol* 155: 3292–3295

118 Sozzani S, Luini W, Borsatti A, Polentarutti N, Zhou D, Piemonti L, D'Amico G, Power CA, Wells TN, Gobbi M, Allavena P, Mantovani A (1997) Receptor expression and

responsiveness of human dendritic cells to a defined set of CC and CXC chemokines. *J Immunol* 159: 1993–2000

119 Caux C, Liu YJ, Banchereau J (1995) Recent advances in the study of dendritic cells and follicular dendritic cells. *Immunol Today* 16: 2–4

120 Sallusto F, Lanzavecchia A (1994) Efficient presentation of soluble antigen by cultured human dendritic cells is maintained by granulocyte/macrophage colony-stimulating factor plus Interleukin-4 and downregulated by tumor necrosis factor-alpha. *J Exp Med* 179: 1109–1118

121 Piemonti L, Bernasconi S, Luini W, Trobonjaca Z, Minty A, Allavena P, Mantovani A (1995) IL-13 supports differentiation of dendritic cells from circulating precursors in concert with GM-CSF. *Eur Cytokine Netw* 6: 245–252

122 Nakamura K, Williams IR, Kupper TS (1995) Keratinocyte-derived monocyte chemoattractant protein 1 (MCP-1): Analysis in a transgenic model demonstrates MCP-1 can recruit dendritic and langerhans cells to skin. *J Invest Dermatol* 105: 635–643

123 Power CA, Church DJ, Meyer A, Alouani S, Proudfoot AEI, Clark-Lewis I, Sozzani S, Mantovani A, Wells TNC (1997) Cloning and characterization of a specific receptor for the novel CC chemokine MIP-3 alpha from lung dendritic cells. *J Exp Med* 186: 825–835

Chemokine receptors

Ingrid U. Schraufstätter[1], Hiroshi Takamori[2] and Robert C. Hoch[1]

[1]Dept. of Immunology, The Scripps Research Institute, 10550 N. Torrey Pines Rd., La Jolla, CA 92037, USA
[2]Dept. of Surgery, Kumamoto University, Kumamoto 860, Japan

Structure of the chemokine receptors

The chemokines exert their influence on target cells via specific G-protein-coupled receptors with seven membrane spanning domains, as predicted by hydropathy plotting. With an estimated 40 to 50 different chemokines, with several of the receptors binding multiple ligands, and with variations in target cell specificity between different species, the individual roles of these receptors are far from clear. More than a dozen putative chemokine receptors have been cloned including several orphan receptors that share sequence homology with the chemokine receptors (reviewed in [1]), but whose ligands are not yet known. These receptors share certain motives such as a DRYLAIV sequence in the second intracellular loop which appears to be involved in G-protein coupling.

Table 1 lists the human chemokine receptors for which specific ligands are known.

Further complicating an understanding of the function of the various receptors comes from an appreciation that receptor expression and usage varies in different species: human neutrophils have similar levels of the two IL-8 receptors (CXCR1 and CXCR2), whereas the rabbit almost exclusively expresses CXCR1 receptors on its neutrophils, and the mouse lacks the CXCR1 as well as IL-8 itself. It seems that different species have developed alternative ways of directing inflammatory cells to their respective destinations.

Studies investigating the importance of specific residues and regions within both the chemokines and their receptors have demonstrated that complex interactions are involved in ligand-receptor binding. This has been most thoroughly explored for IL-8 receptors and their ligands, which may serve as a paradigm for studies of other chemokine-receptor interactions. The two human IL-8 receptors, designated CXCR1 (or IL-8 receptor A in the older literature), and CXCR 2 (IL-8 receptor B), have primary sequences that are 77% identical [2, 3], differing most notably in their extracellular N-terminal domains and in the intracellular C-terminus, and to a lesser degree in the second extracellular loop and adjacent transmembrane domains. The

Table 1 - Human chemokine receptors and their ligands

Receptor	Ligands
CCR1	MIP-1α, RANTES, MCP-3
CCR2	MCP-1, MCP-3, MCP-5
CCR3	Eotaxin, RANTES, MCP-2, MCP-3
CCR4	MIP-1α, RANTES, MCP-1, TARC
CCR5	MIP-1α, MIP-1β, RANTES
CCR6	LARC
CCR7	ELC
CCR8	I-309
CXCR1	IL-8
CXCR2	IL-8, GRO-α, GRO-β, GRO-γ, NAP-2, ENA-78
CXCR3	IP10, MIG
CXCR4	SDF-1

CXCR1 possesses great ligand specificity, binding to IL-8 with high affinity ($K_d \sim 1$ to 2 nM), but binding with low affinity (>100 nM) to the IL-8 related chemoattractant proteins melanoma growth stimulating activity (MGSA/GRO-α) and neutrophil activating peptide 2 (NAP-2), whereas CXCR2 exhibits less specifity in ligand interaction, binding not only to IL-8 ($K_d \sim 1$ to 2 nM), but also to MGSA ($K_d \sim 1$ to 2 nM), NAP-2 ($K_d \sim 2$ to 5 nM) and ENA78 ($K_d \sim 1$ to 2 nM) with high affinity [4, 5].

It has been shown that the Glu^4-Leu^5-Arg^6 sequence in the N-terminal region of IL-8 is necessary for high-affinity binding to the neutrophil [6, 19]. This sequence is conserved in the neutrophil-stimulating members of the chemokine family and is a prerequisite for the binding of MGSA and NAP-2 to CXCR2. Peptides containing the Glu-Leu-Arg sequence were, however, not capable of binding to or activating the IL-8 receptors, and a mutant of IL-8 in which the Glu-Leu-Arg sequence was replaced with alanines could still activate both the CXCR1 and CXCR2, when added in high concentrations. In lower concentrations these mutant CXC chemokines, especially those in which the Glu-Leu-Arg sequence was replaced with Ala-Ala-Arg, became antagonists [7, 8].

Additional binding regions of IL-8 seem to differ for the CXCR1 and CXCR2, and possibly also vary for the different CXC chemokines that bind to the CXCR2. In the case of the CXCR1, a zone between Cys^7 and Cys^{50} was identified as a second binding region [9]. Subsequently, it was demonstrated that Tyr^{13}-Ser^{14}-Lys^{15} within this region are important for high affinity binding to this receptor [10]. Phe^{21} and Leu^{49} also contribute to high affinity binding to the CXCR1, forming a surface accessible hydrophobic cluster with Tyr[13] and Ser[14] [11]. Interestingly, the loop region around Tyr[13]-Ser[14]-Lys[15] in IL-8 is the area of the greatest structural difference between IL-8 and MGSA. Replacing the MGSA sequence with the corresponding amino acids of IL-8 (Ile[10] to Phe[17]) increases its affinity for the CXCR1 by an order of magnitude with little effect on CXCR2 binding [12]. If, in addition to this sequence replacement Phe[21] and Leu[49] – the two amino acids in IL-8 that form a binding pocket with Tyr[13]-Ser[14] – are expressed on an MGSA background, the chimeric construct reaches an affinity of 1-2 nM with both receptors [12]. Taken together these results define a second binding region of IL-8 for CXCR1, which comprises Tyr[13], Ser[14], Phe[21] and Leu[49].

A region of IL-8, in addition to ELR, required for high-affinity binding to CXCR2 was found to lie in the carboxy-terminal α-helix [9]. This α-helix also seems to play a role in binding of NAP-2 and the mouse equivalent of IL-8, N51 [13]. Within this region no specific amino acids that are important for binding have been defined.

The three-dimensional structure of IL-8 [14] shows a distance of 20 to 25 Å between the N-terminal ELR and either the Tyr[13]-Ser[14] region or the carboxy-terminal α-helix, which implies multiple binding sites on the IL-8 receptors.

Initial experiments indicated that the N-terminus of the receptor determines whether it behaves like the CXCR1, which specifically recognizes IL-8, or like the CXCR2, which also binds MGSA and NAP-2 with high affinity [15, 16]. Furthermore this area appears to recognize the Tyr[13]-Ser[14]-Lys[15] region on IL-8, which together with ELR has been found to be essential for high-affinity binding to the CXCR1 [10]. These results, all obtained by binding of ligand to chimeric receptors expressed in mammalian cell lines, were further supported by NMR analysis of complexes formed between IL-8 and the first 40 amino acids of the CXCR1, which indicated binding of this receptor stretch to the clustered second binding site including Tyr[13] and Lys[15] [17]. In addition, a synthetic peptide representing amino acids 9 to 29 of the receptor blocks IL-8 binding to the CXCR1 with a Ki of 13 μM [18]. This ligand/receptor interaction is, however, not sufficient for ligand binding and/or receptor activation: Chimeric receptor constructs that switch from either of the two IL-8 receptors to the formyl peptide receptor in the first transmembrane domain are dysfunctional. Thus it is not surprising that amino acids in the second and third extracellular loops of the IL-8 receptors were found to be crucial for high affinity ligand binding. Using point mutated CXCR1 constructs, Arg[199] and Arg[203] of the second extracellular loop, and Asp[265], Glu[275] and Arg[280] of the third extracellular loop were found to be essential for high affinity ligand binding [19, 20]. The corresponding third extracellular loop amino acids on the CXCR2 (Glu[279] and Arg[284]) were similarly important for IL-8 and MGSA high affinity binding. The Arg[284] to Ala CXCR2 mutant responded equally well to an IL-8 mutant in which the Glu[4]-Leu[5]-Arg[6] sequence was replaced with alanines as to wild type IL-8, implying that this part of the third extracellular loop of the IL-8 receptors binds to the Glu-Leu-

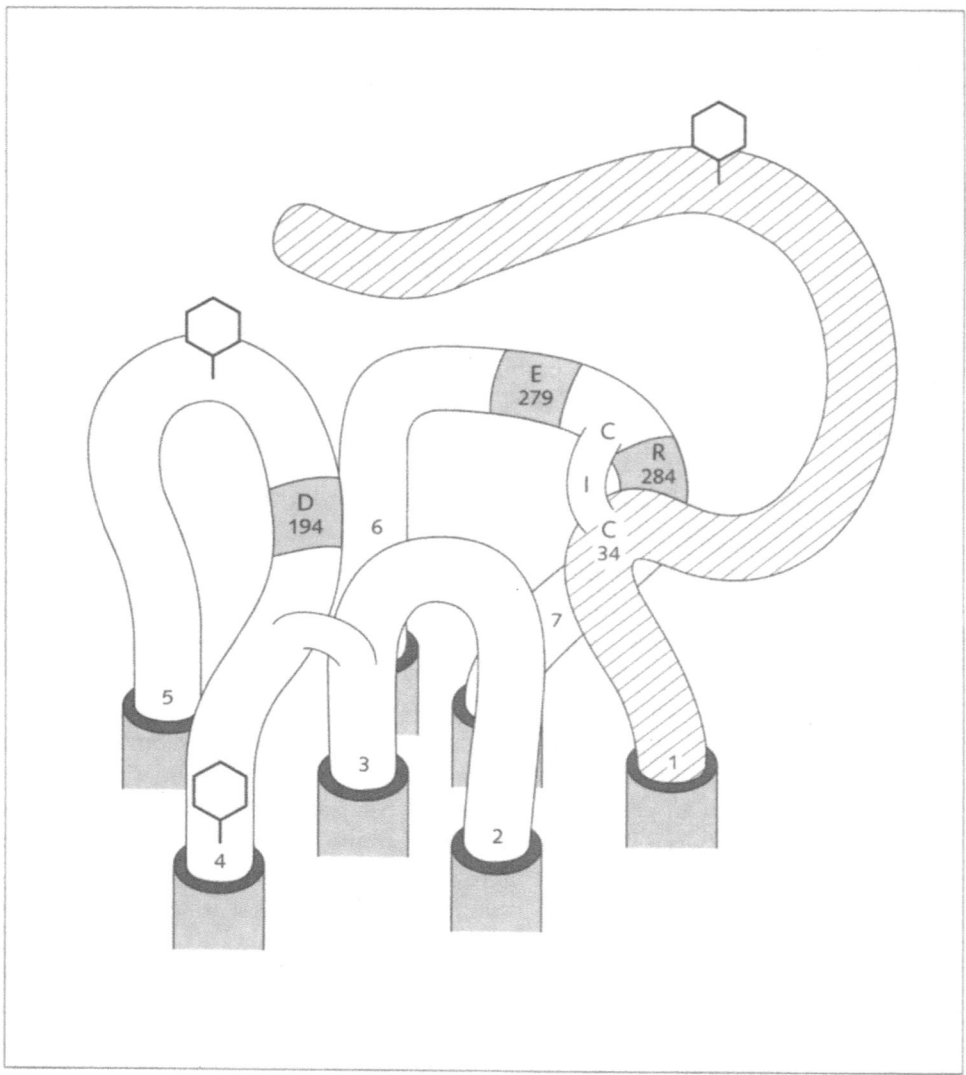

Figure 1

Model of the proposed structure of the ligand binding domains of the CXCR2. Proposed binding sites are shaded. The transmembrane domains (1–7) have been arranged according to the distribution using the low resolution x-ray diffraction results for rhodopsin and a computer based arrangement of their distribution in G-protein coupled receptors generally. Disulfide bridges and the location of the ELR binding site of the receptor correspond to the model proposed for the CXCR1. The second proposed binding site on the second extracellular loop is unique to the CXCR2.

Arg sequence of IL-8 (Schraufstätter et al., unpublished results). Replacement of the second extracellular loop of the CXCR2 with CXCR1 sequence led to a 60-fold lower affinity for IL-8. This loss in affinity could be ascribed to a single amino acid: If Asp^{194} was replaced with the corresponding amino acid in the CXCR1, a valine, the affinity was similarly 50 to 60-fold decreased. Figure 1 shows a model for the binding of IL-8 to the CXCR2.

The complexity of the binding behavior may explain why screening for small molecular weight antagonists for IL-8 has been difficult. It may be necessary to combine inhibitors that react at different sites of interaction. As mentioned above several peptide inhibitors have been described [18, 7, 21] which block IL-8 activation in the 10 μM range. It may also be possible to dissociate receptor binding from receptor activation as described recently for an antibody to the CXCR1 [22].

Less is known about the binding domains of the CC receptors, which have only been cloned during the last few years, but there is little doubt that their ligand/receptor interactions are similarly complicated. Chimeric constructs between the CCR1 and CCR2 indicated that the receptor amino terminus is important for binding of MCP-1 to the CCR2, but not for binding of MIP-1α to the CCR1 [23]. The same amino terminal CCR2 receptor domain followed by CCR5 receptor sequence allows binding of both MCP-1 and MIP-1α, but in contrast to the full length CCR5 does not function as a coreceptor for the entry of macrophage tropic strains of HIV [24].

A number of chemokine receptors allow the entry of viruses into cells: In addition to the just mentioned CCR5, HIV infection is also supported by the CXCR4 [25, 26] and the newly cloned orphan receptors BOB and Bonzo [27, 28].

Other viruses encode chemokine receptor-like molecules themselves: *Herpesvirus saimiri*'s ECRF resembles the CXCRs and like the CXCR2 binds IL-8, MGSA and NAP-2 [29]. The herpes virus isolated from Kaposi's sarcoma lesions also encodes an IL-8 binding chemokine receptor [30]. Interestingly, this receptor is constitutively active and may be involved in transforming the infected cell in Kaposi's sarcoma [31]. A human cytomegalovirus encoded sequence binds several CC chemokines [32].

The only receptor that binds both CC and CXC chemokines is the Duffy antigen receptor for chemokines (DARC) [33], originally identified as a red blood cell antigen, important for the entry of *Plasmodium vivax*, but also present on postcapillary endothelial cells [34]. It is questionable to call this molecule a receptor, since it has not been shown to transduct any signal when it binds ligand. It is not known whether this receptor functions as a sink for chemokines or as a docking receptor which presents chemokines to circulating leukocytes.

Function of the chemokine receptors

As do other neutrophilic stimuli, IL-8 induces numerous functional responses in PMNs including Ca^{2+} mobilization, cytoskeletal rearrangement, chemotaxis, and phagocytosis (all reviewed in [35–37]), but only limited granule secretion and minimal release of superoxide anion. Thus IL-8 appears to be a powerful chemoattractant without initiating much oxidative damage on its own.

Similarly, the CC chemokines cause Ca^{2+} mobilization and attraction of lymphocytes or monocytes, but cause little tissue damage by themselves. For instance, mice that express the murine MCP-1 under control of an insulin promotor show pronounced monocytic insulinitis, but no signs of pancreatic tissue damage or diabetes [38].

The role of chemokines *in vivo* is certainly more complex than mere leukocyte attraction, however. High concentrations of IL-8 have been found in many acute and chronic inflammatory diseases from ARDS [39] to rheumatoid arthritis and psoriasis [40]. In addition, antibodies to IL-8 have proved beneficial in several animal models of acute inflammation [41–43].

While IL-8 itself causes massive neutrophil attraction without immediately causing tissue injury, small concentration of formylated peptides and C5a – both of which present at sites of bacterial infection – are capable of activating the respiratory burst, and even a neutrophil which is not activated will release its enzymes into the surrounding tissue as it dies over the next 24 h.

In cells that express the correct G-protein, binding to either of the two IL-8 receptors induces calcium translocation and actin polymerization, as evidenced by experiments evaluating these receptors individually in transfected cell lines [44, 45]. In the neutrophil IL-8 receptor activation is inhibited by pertussis toxin [46] which inactivates the $Gi\alpha s$. More recently, it has been shown that the IL-8 receptors in the neutrophil couple to $Gi\alpha_2$ [47], a response that depends on the second intracellular loop as well as the membrane adjacent area of the COOH-terminus. The receptors are, however, capable of transferring their signal through $G\alpha_{16}$ in cells in which this G-protein is abundant [48].

CC receptors are also inhibited by pertussis toxin, which is indicative of $Gi\alpha$ coupling, but depending on the cell type in which they are expressed, CC receptors can also couple to $G\alpha q$, a response that depends on the third intracellular loop [49].

The exact mechanism of the receptor/G protein interaction is not understood for any of the G-proteins, but seems to involve receptor sequences of only a few amino acids.

Phosphorylation of G-protein coupled receptors leads to their desensitization and internalization. For the chemokine receptors this phosphorylation process appears to occur primarily on the COOH terminus. In the case of the CXCR2, phosphorylation occurs within 10 to 20 s following the addition of IL-8 and is limited to phosphorylation of serines 348 and possibly 346 (see Fig. 2). These rapid kinetics of receptor inactivation may help to explain the transiency of the cellular response to IL-8, which seems to shut down within the amount of time that is necessary to assemble the molecules for the respiratory burst.

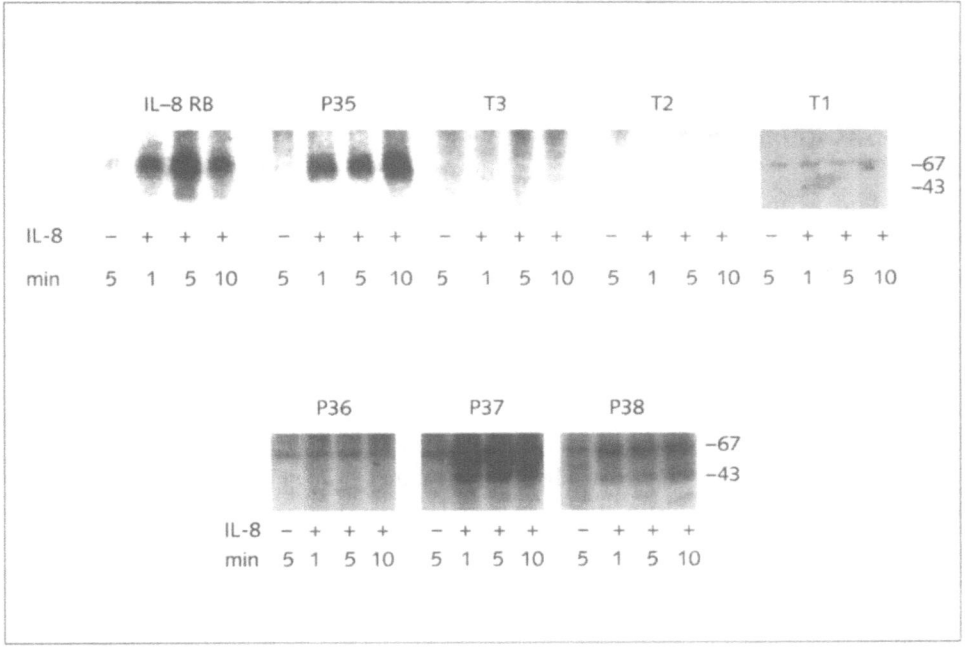

Figure 2
Phosphorylation of CXCR2 mutants in RBL2H3 cells: RBL2H3 cells expressing wild type CXCR2 or receptor mutants were [32P]-phosphate labelled, stimulated with 10⁻⁷M IL-8 for 1 to 10 min and immunoprecipitated with polyclonal rabbit anti-CXCR2 antibody[61].The autorad exposure for P35 and CXCR2 was 24 h, and for T3 36 h to verify the absence of specific label in these cells. T2 and T1 similarly showed no phosphorylation. The bottom panel shows a 60-h exposure of single amino acid substitution mutants. P38 was poorly and belatedly phosphorylated, P37 behaved like wild type receptor, while no phosphorylation could be detected on P36.

-RHGLLKILAIHGLISKD				T1
-RHGLLKILAIHGLISKDSLPKD				T2
-RHGLLKILAIHGLISKDSLPKDSRPSF				T3
-RHGLLKILAIHGLISKDSLPKDSRPSFVGSSSGHNANAL				P35
-RHGLLKILAIHGLISKDSLPKDSRPSFVGASSGHTSTTL				P36
- RHGLLKILAIHGLISKDSLPKDSRPSFVGSASGHTSTTL				P37
-RHGLLKILAIHGLISKDSLPKDSRPSFVGSSAGHTSTTL				P38
-RHGLLKILAIHGLISKDSLPKDSRPSFVGSSSGHTSTTL				wild type
320	330	340	350	

Although either the CXCR1 or the CXCR2 may mediate neutrophil activation, these receptors may not be equally important in affecting neutrophil chemotaxis. Neutralizing antibodies to the CXCR1 largely prevent (70% to 80%) neutrophil chemotaxis *in vitro* in response to IL-8 [50, 51], whereas neutralizing antibodies to the CXCR2 inhibit IL-8 induced chemotaxis only by 20% to 30%, suggesting that CXCR1 may be relatively more important than CXCR2 in mediating IL-8 induced neutrophil chemotaxis, even though both receptors were found to be expressed in roughly equal numbers on the surface of the human neutrophils, as assessed by fluorescence-activated cell sorting technique. One may speculate that the faster phosphorylation and desensitization observed for the CXCR2 may render the CXCR1 more effective in processes that involve prolonged activation such as chemotaxis.

IL-8 receptors are not only found on leukocytes, but also on melanoma cells [52, 53], some lung cancer cell lines and transformed keratinocytes. All of these cells produce both IL-8 and MGSA themselves, which function as autocrine growth factors for these cells. Furthermore, the Glu-Leu-Arg containing CXC chemokines are angiogenic factors that promote tumor metastasis [54, 55], while the CXC chemokines lacking this sequence appear angiostatic [56]. Considering the ligand affinity of the CXCR2 for all of the Glu-Leu-Arg containing chemokines, one may speculate that their angiogenic effect depends on the presence of the CXCR2 on the endothelium, but it has been impossible so far to detect this receptor on cultured endothelial cells. This finding may be due to the absence of receptor expression on cultures endothelium and/or down-regulation of surface expression of CXCR by endogenously produced ligands. Nevertheless, immunohistochemistry has identified CXCR2 presence on endothelium at the margins of debrided burn wounds in areas of rapid tissue proliferation [57]. Specific gene induction and/or the presence of the physiological milieu of surrounding cells and cell matrix may be important for this phenomenon, which so far eludes explanation.

It is intriguing to speculate that lymphocyte trafficking to specific sites may be mediated by specific chemokine receptors on these cells. BLR-1, for instance, a B-cell receptor with homology to the CCRs is necessary for the development of germinal centers in secondary follicles in the spleen [58]. Expression of chemokine receptors also appears to be important for hematopoeisis and release of leukocytes from the bone marrow [59, 60].

No doubt, many questions have not been answered yet, but the importance of chemokine receptors for leukocyte attraction with its inflammatory sequelae and for increased cell growth in cancers as well as during chronic inflammatory disease seem to be well documented.

References

1   Rollins, BJ (1997) Chemokines. *Blood* 90: 909–928
2   Holmes W, Lee J, Kuang WJ, Rice G, Wood W (1991) Structure and functional expression of a human interleukin-8 receptor. *Science* 253: 1278–1280
3   Murphy P, Tiffany H (1991) Cloning of complimentary DNA encoding a functional human IL-8 receptor. *Science* 2531280–1283
4   Lee J, Horuk R, Rice GC, Bennett GL, Camerato T, Wood WI (1992) Characterization of two high affinity human interleukin-8 receptors. *J Biol Chem* 267: 16283–16287
5   Bozic C.R, Gerard N. P, Gerard C (1996) Receptor binding specificity and pulmonary gene expression of the neutrophil-activating peptide ENA-78. *Am J Respir Cell Mol Biol* 14: 302–308
6   Clark-Lewis I, Schumacher C, Baggiolini M, Moser B (1991) Structure-activity relationships for interleukin-8 determined using chemically synthesized analogs. Critical role of NH2-terminal residues and evidence for uncoupling of neutrophil chemotaxis, exocytosis, and receptor binding affinities. *J Biol Chem* 266: 23128–23134
7   Moser B, Dewald B, Barella L, Schumacher C, Baggiolini M, Clark-Lewis I (1993) Interleukin-8 antagonists generated by N-terminal modification. *J Biol Chem* 268: 7125–7128
8   Zagorski J, Wahl SM (1997) Inhibition of acute peritoneal inflammation in rats by a cytokine-induced neutrophil chemoattractant receptor antagonist. *J Immunol* 159: 1059–1062
9   Schraufstätter IU, Barrett DS, Ma M, Oades ZG, Cochrane, CG (1993) Multiple sites on IL-8 responsible for binding to a and b IL-8 Receptors. *J Immunol* 151: 6418–6428
10 Schraufstätter IU, Ma M, Oades ZG, Barrett DS, Cochrane CG (1995) The role of tyr13 and lys15 of IL-8 in the high affinity interaction with the A receptor. *J Biol Chem* 270: 10428–10431
11 Hammond MEW, Shyamala V, Siani MA, Gallegos CA, Feucht PH, Abbott J, Lapointe GR, Moghadam M, Khoja H, Zakel J, Tekamp-Olsen P (1996) Receptor recognition and specificity of interleukin-8 is determined by residues that cluster near a surface-accessible hydrophobic pocket. *J Biol Chem* 271: 8228–8235
12 Lowman HB, Slagle P H, DeForge LE, Wirth CM, Gillece-Castro BL, Bourell JH, Fairbrother WJ (1996) Exchanging interleukin-8 and melanoma growth-stimulating activity receptor binding specificities. *J Biol Chem* 271: 14344–14352
13 Heinrich JN, O'Rourke E, Chen L, Gray H, Dorfman KS Bravo R (1994) Biological activity of the growth factor-induced cytokine N51: Structure-function analysis using N51/interleukin-8 chimeric molecules. *Mol Cell Biol* 14: 2849–2861
14 Clore G, Appella E, Yamada M, Matsushima K, Gronenborn A (1990) Three-dimensional structure of IL-8 in solution. *Biochemistry* 29: 1689–1696
15 LaRosa GJ, Thomas K, Kaufmann ME, Mark R,White M, Taylor L, Gray G, Witt D, Navarro J (1992) Amino terminus of the interleukin-8 receptor is a major determinant of receptor subtype specificity. *J Biol Chem* 267: 25402–25406

16   Gayle RB, Sleath P, Srinivason S, Birks CW, Weerawarna KS, Cerretti DP, Kozlosky KJ, Nelson N, Vanden Bos T, Beckmann MP (1993) Importance of the amino terminus of the interleukin-8 receptor in ligand interaction. *J Biol Chem* 286: 7283–7289

17   Clubb RT, Omichinski J, Clore GM, Gronenborn AM (1994) Mapping the binding surface of interleukin-8 complexes with an N-terminal fragment of the type 1 human interleukin-8 receptor. *Febs Lett* 338: 93–97

18   Attwood MR, Borkakoti N, Bottomley GA, Conway EA, Cowan I, Fallowfield AG, Handa BK, Jones PS, Keech E, Kirtland SJ, Williams G, Wilson FX (1996) Identification and characterization of an inhibitor of interleukin-8: A receptor based approach. *Bioorg Med Chem Let* 6: 1869–1874

19   Hébert C, Chuntharapai A, Smith M, Colby T, Kim J, Horuk R (1993) Partial functional mapping of the human interleukin-8 type A receptor. *J Biol Chem* 268: 18549–18553

20   Leong SR, Kabakoff R, Hebert CA (1994) Complete mutagenesis of the extracellular domain of interleukin-8 (IL-8) Type A receptor identifies charged residues mediating IL-8 binding and signal transduction. *J Biol Chem* 269: 19343–19348

21   Hayashi S, Kurdowska A, Miller EJ, Albright ME, Girten BE, Cohen AB (1995) Synthetic hexa- and heptapeptides which inhibit IL-8 from binding to and activating human blood neutrophils. *J Immunol* 154: 814–824

22   Wu L, Ruffing N, Shi X, Newman W, Soler D, Mackay CR, Qin S (1996) Discrete steps in binding and signaling of interleukin-8 with its receptor. *J Biol Chem* 271: 31202–31207

23   Monteclaro FS, Charo IF (1996) The amino-terminal extracellular domain of the MCP-1 receptor, but not the RANTES/MIP-1a receptor, confers chemokine selectivity. *J Biol Chem* 271: 19084–19092

24   Farzan M, Choe H, Martin KA, Sun Y, Sidelko M, Mackay CR, Gerard NP, Sodroski J, Gerard C (1997) HIV-1 entry and macrophage inflammatory protein-1b-mediated signaling are independent functions of the chemokine receptor CCR5). *J Biol Chem* 272: 6854–6857

25   Oberlin E, Amara A, Bachelerie F, Bessia C, Virelizier JL, Arenzana-Seisdedos F, Schwartz O, Heard JM, Clark-Lewis I, Legler DF, Loetscher M, Baggiolini M, Moser B (1996) The CXC chemokine SDF-1 is the ligand for LESTR/fusin and prevents infection by T-cell-line adapted HIV-1). *Nature* 382: 833–835

26   Bleul CC, Farzan M, Choe H, Parolin C, Clark-Lewis I, Sodroski J, Springer TA (1996) The lymphocyte chemoattractant SDF-1 is a ligand for LESTR/fusin and blocks HIV-1 entry. *Nature* 382: 829–833

27   Liao F, Alkhatib G, Peden KWC, Sharma G, Berger EA, Farber JM (1997) STRL33, a novel chemokine receptor-like protein, functions as a fusion cofactor for both macrophage-tropic and T-cell line-tropic HIV-1). *J Exp Med* 185: 2015–2023

28   Deng H, Unutmaz D, Kewal Ramani VN, and Littman DR (1997) Expression cloning of new receptors used by simian and human immunodeficiency viruses. *Nature* 388: 296–300

29   Ahuja SK, Murphy P (1993) Molecular piracy of mammalian Interleukin-8 receptor Type B by *Herpesvirus Saimiri*. *J Biol Chem* 268: 20691–20694

30   Cesarman E, Nador R G, Bai F, Bohenzky RA, Russo JJ, Moore PS, Chang Y, Knowles DM (1996) Kaposi's sarcoma-associated herpesvirus contains G protein-coupled receptor and cyclin D homologs which are expressed in Kaposi's sarcoma and maligant lymphoma. *J Virol* 70: 8218–8223

31   Arvanitakis L, Geras-Raaka E, Varma A, Gershengorn MC, Cesarman E (1997) Human herpesvirus KSHV encodes a constitutively active G-protein-coupled receptor linked to cell proliferation. *Nature* 385: 347–350

32   Gao JL, Murphy PM (1994) Human cytomegalovirus open reading frame US28 encodes a functional beta chemokine receptor. *J Biol Chem* 269: 28539–28544

33   Horuk R, Chitnis C E, Darbonne WC, Colby TJ, Rybicki A, Hadley TJ, Miller LH (1993) A receptor for the malarial parasite plasmodium vivax: the erythrocyte chemokine receptor. *Science* 261: 1182–1184

34   Hadley TR, Lu Z, Wasniowska K, Martin AW, Peiper SC, Hesselgesser J, Horuk R (1994) Postcapillary venule endothelial cells in kidney express a multispecific chemokine receptor that is structurally and functionally identical to the erythroid Isoform, which is the Duffy blood group antigen. *J Clin Invest* 94: 985–991

35   Matsushima K, Baldwin E, Mukaida N (1992) Interleukin-8 and MCAF: novel leukocyte recruitment and activating cytokines. *Chem Immunol* 51: 236–265

36   Baggiolini M, Walz A, Kunkel S (1989) Neutrophil activating peptide/interleukin 8, a novel cytokine that activates neutrophils. *J Clin Invest* 84: 1045–1049

37   Hébert C, Baker J (1993) Interleukin-8: a review. *Cancer Invest* 11: 743–750

38   Greval IS, Rutledge J, Fiorello JA, Gu L, Gladue RP, Flavell RA, Rollins BJ (1997) Transgenic monocyte attractant protein-1 (MCP-1) in pancreatic islets produces monocyte-rich insulitis without diabetes: Abrogation by a second transgene expressing systemic MCP-1). *J Immunol* 159: 401–409

39   Goodman RB, Strieter RM, Steinberg KP, Milberg JA, Maunder RJ, Kunkel SL, Walz A, Hudson LD, Martin TR (1995) Correlation of BALF cytokine levels with inflammatory cell populations in ARDS. *Am J Resp Crit Care Med* 151: A78

40   Schröder J, Mrowietz U, Morita E, Christophers E (1987) Purification and partial biochemical characterization of a human monocyte-derived, neutrophil activating peptide that lacks interleukin 1 activity. *J Immunol* 139: 3474–3483

41   Broaddus VC, Boylan A, Hoeffel JM, Kim KJ, Sadick M, Chuntharapai A, Hebert CA (1994) Neutralization of IL-8 inhibits neutrophil influx in a rabbit model of endotoxin-induced pleurisy. *J Immunol* 152: 2960–2967

42   Folkesson HG , Matthay MA, Hebert CA, Broaddus VC (1995) Acid aspiration-induced lung injury in rabbits is mediated by interleukin-8-dependent mechanisms. *J Clin Invest* 96: 107–116

43   Sekido N, Mukaida N, Harada A, Nakanishi I, Watanabe Y, Matsushima K (1993) Prevention of lung reperfusion injury in rabbits by monoclonal antibody against interleukin-8. *Nature* 365: 655–657

44 Norgauer J, Krutmann J, Dobos GJ, Traynor-Kaplan AE, Oades ZG, Schraufstätter IU (1994) Actin polymerization, calcium-transients, and phospholipid metabolism in human neutrophils after stimulation with interleukin-8 and N-formyl peptide. *J Invest Dermatol* 102: 310–314

45 Ahuja SK, Lee JC, Murphy PM (1996) CXC chemokines bind to unique sets of selectivity determinants that can function independentlt and are broadly distributed on multiple domains of human interleukin-8 receptor B. *J Biol Chem* 271: 225–22

46 Thelen M, Peveri P, Kernen P, von Tscharner V, Walz A, Baggiolini M (1988) Mechanism of neutrophil activation by NAF, a novel monocyte-derived peptide antagonist *FASEB J* 2: 2702–2706

47 Damaj BB, McColl S R, Mahana W, Crouch MF, Naccache PH (1996) Physical association of G_{i2a} with interleukin-8 receptors. *J Biol Chem* 271: 12783–12789

48 Wu D, LaRosa G J, Simon MI (1993) G-protein-coupled signal transduction pathways for interleukin-8. *Science* 261: 101–103

49 Arai H, Charo IF (1996) Differential regulation of G-protein-mediated signaling by chemokine receptors. *J Biol Chem* 271: 21814–21819

50 Chuntharapai A, Lee J, Hebert CA, Kim KJ (1994) Monoclonal antibodies detect different distribution patterns of IL-8 receptor A and IL-8 receptor B on human peripheral blood leukocytes. *J Immunol* 153: 5682–5688

51 Hammond MEW, Lapointe GR, Feucht PH, Hilt S, Gallegos CA, Gordon CA, Giedlin MA, Mullenbach G, Tekamp-Olsen P (1995) IL-8 induces neutrophil chemotaxis predominantly via type I IL-8 receptors. *J Immunol* 155: 1428–1433

52 Richmond A, Balantien H, Thomas H, Flaggs G, Barton D, Spiess J, Bordoni R, Francke U, Derynck R (1989) Molecular characterization of melanoma growth stimulatory activity, a growth factor structurally related to β-thromboglobulin. *EMBO J* 7: 2025–2033

53 Norgauer J, Metzner B, Schraufstätter I (1996) Expression and growth-promoting function of the IL-8 receptor b in human melanoma cells. *J Immunol* 156:

54 Koch AE, Polverini P, Kunkel SL, Harlow LA, DiPietro LA, Elner VM, Elner SG, Strieter RM (1992) Interleukin-8 as a macrophage-derived mediator of angiogenesis. *Science* 258: 1798–1801

55 Arenberg DA, Kunkel S L, Polverini PJ, Glass M, Burdick MD, Strieter RM (1996) Inhibition of interleukin-8 reduces tumorigenesis of human non-small cell lung cancer in SCID mice. *J Clin Invest* 97: 2792–2802

56 Strieter RM, Polverini PJ, Kunkel S L, Arenberg DA, Burdick D, Kasper J, Dzuiba J, Van Dame J, Walz A, Marriott D, Chan SY, Roczniak S, Shanafel AB (1995) The functional role of the ELR motif in CXC chemokine-mediated angiogenesis. *J Biol Chem* 270: 27348–27357

57 Nanney LB, Mueller SG, Bueno R, Peiper SC, Richmond A (1995) Distributions of melanoma growth stimulatory activity of growth-regulated gene and the interleukin-8 receptor in human wound repair. *Am J Pathol* 147: 1248–1260

58 Förster R, Mattis AE, Kremmer E, Wolf E, Brem G, Lipp M (1996) A putative chemo-

kine receptor, BLR1, directs B cell migration to defined lymphoid organs and specific anatomic compartments of teh spleen. *Cell* 87: 1037–1047

59 Broxmeyer HE, Sherry B, Cooper S, Lu L, Maze R, Beckmann MP, Cerami A, Ralph P (1993) Comparative analysis of the human macrophage inflammatory protein family of cytokines (chemokines) on proliferation of human myeloid progenitor cells Interacting effects involving suppression, synergistic suppression, and blocking of suppression. *J Immunol* 150: 3448–3455

60 Cacalano G, Lee J, Kikly K, Ryan AM, Pitts-Meek S, Hultgren B, Wood WI, Moore MW (1994) Neutrophil and B cell expansion in mice that lack the murine IL-8 receptor homolog. *Nature* 265: 682–684

61 Norgauer J, Metzner B, Schraufstätter I (1996) Expression and growth promoting function of the IL-8 receptor B in human melanoma cells. *J Immunol* 156: 1132–1137

Regulation of gene expression of chemokines and their receptors

Hans Sprenger[1], Andreas Kaufmann[2], Delia Bussfeld[2], and Diethard Gemsa[2]

[1]Institute of Laboratory Medicine, Leopoldina-Hospital, Gustav-Adolf-Str. 8,
D-97422 Schweinfurt, Germany
[2]Institute of Immunology, Philipps-University Marburg, Robert-Koch-Str. 17,
D-35037 Marburg, Germany

Introduction

Over the past decades, at an ever-accelerating pace, numerous members of a new family of cytokines with leukocyte attracting and activating properties, called chemotactic cytokines (chemokines), have been identified. Chemokines are highly regulated proteins of low molecular mass (5–15 kD, 70–80 amino acids) that have to be considered as the main chemotactic factors responsible for the recruitment of distinct effector cells to sites of tissue injury and inflammation. The site-directed immigration of leukocytes is provoked by gradients of chemokines immobilized to extracellular matrix components [1]. In addition, chemokines contribute to vascular adhesion and promote transendothelial migration [2, 3]. The position of the first two cysteins and the presence or absence of an ELR-motif preceding the first cystein, have been used to subdivide the chemokine family into at least five branches, including the recently defined C- and CX_3C-branches. Chemokines are inducible in a wide variety of different tissues by many stimuli such as mechanical injury, bacteria, viruses, bacterially or virally derived molecules and finally by many proinflammatory cytokines. The most abundant inducible mRNAs found in activated T cells seem to be chemokines (reviewed in [4]). All chemokines so far identified, have been found to bind to G-protein coupled receptors featuring seven hydrophobic transmembrane domains. Most chemokine receptors are not specific for only one ligand, but can promiscuously bind to different chemokines of the same branch with varying affinities. The exception is the Duffy antigen receptor on erythrocytes which binds to a wide variety of CC- as well as CXC-chemokines and does not signal via G-proteins. The structure, induction, and biological activities of chemokines and chemokine-receptors have been summarized in several recent comprehensive reviews [5–10]. However, a comprehensive summary of recently published gene regulatory mechanisms is still lacking. This review will focus on the regulated gene expression of chemokines and their receptors, with special emphasis on inflammatory processes.

Chemokines and Skin, edited by E. Kownatzki and J. Norgauer
© 1998 Birkhäuser Verlag Basel/Switzerland

Chemokines

Chemokine expression after mechanical injury

ELR-CXC-chemokines have been shown to participate in tissue remodeling, repair, wound healing [11, 12], and neovascularization [13]. Mere cellular detachment or deformation is a sufficient stimulus for IL-8 gene expression [14]. In particular, IL-8 and GRO were found to be angiogenic [13] while non-ELR-CXC-chemokines such as IP-10 tend to have a rather anti-angiogenic effect [15, 16] by binding to a specific cell surface heparan sulfate site on endothelial cells [17]. For IL-8, no such binding sites have been identified to date, and the molecular mechanisms of chemokine interaction with endothelial cells is controversial [18, 19]. In contrast to the general angiogenic properties of ELR-CXC-chemokines, GRO-α and -β have been reported to inhibit angiogenesis so that the general importance of this model is questionable [20].

Proteins of the phylogenetically bacteria-derived mitochondria are N-formylated and, like formyl-peptides (e.g. fMLP) of bacteriae, act as chemoattractants for neutrophils [21]. Thus, mitochondria from damaged tissue may provide a first signal to attract phagocytes initiating repair processes.

Chemokines induced by bacteria, viruses, and bacterially and virally derived molecules

Chemokine gene expression differs substantially with respect to tissue specific inducibility and kinetics of production. Stimulated monocytes and macrophages are a major source of various chemokines. LPS derived from the cell wall of gramnegative bacteria is known to be a strong macrophage activator and induces the rapid release of most CXC- as well as CC-chemokines. This is not applicable to viral infections. Exposure of human monocytes to influenza A virus has been shown to selectively induce mononuclear cell attracting chemokines whereas, in striking contrast, the expression of neutrophil attracting chemokines was suppressed as long as no bacterially-derived products such as LPS were present [22]. Our particular interest in the role of CC-chemokines in antiviral defense is supported by other recent studies: MIP-1α has to be considered a major monocyte and lymphocyte chemoattractant as shown by previous *in vivo* studies performed in a MIP-1α-deficient mouse model [23]. The general importance of CC-chemokines has recently been underlined by their apparent anti-HIV avtivity [24]. The induction of mononuclear leukocyte attracting chemokines after virus infection has been previously reported for MCP-1 and MCP-2 after exposure of monocytes to measles virus [25] and for IP-10 in astrocytes and microglia by Newcastle disease virus [26]. The minimal response element for both measles virus- and IFN-γ-induced IP-10 expression has been shown to consist of an IFN-stimulated response element (ISRE) and a NF-κB-site [27]. Besides an indirect induction via virus-induced IFN, IP-10 expression seems to be directly upregulated by virus infection, independent of a primary IFN-response ([27] and our own unpublished observations). However, only a few attempts have been undertaken to identify viral key molecules and the basic mechanisms involved in the regulation of chemokine gene expression.

Rather contradictory results have been published for the viral inducibility of the neutrophil attracting chemokine IL-8. Measles virus has been reported to induce IL-8 in fibroblasts [28] and influenza A virus, respiratory syncytial virus (RSV) and rhinovirus in pulmonary epithelial cells [29–31]. In contrast, recent reports demonstrate RSV to suppress IL-8 production by induction of IL-10 [32], and IL-8 gene transcription has been shown to be inhibited by virus-inducible interferon [33]. Our results clearly support the notion that an exposure to influenza A virus, regardless of whether it is live or inactivated, does not induce the production of neutrophil attracting CXC-chemokines and instead selectively induces mononuclear cell attracting chemokines. The differences from previous reports [28-31] may be explained by the easy inducibility of the IL-8 gene. Even adherence [34] or detachment [14] of cells represent sufficient stimuli for the upregulation of IL-8 expression.

Regulation of chemokine gene expression by proinflammatory cytokines

Principally, chemokines are secondary mediators that are inducible by primary proinflammatory cytokines such as TNF and IL-1 (reviewed in [5, 6], Fig. 1) by means of transcriptional activation and posttranscriptional increase of mRNA-stability. However, a primary induction of chemokine expression, for example, upon contact with bacteria or bacteria-derived products, has at least been shown in cells of the monocyte/macrophage lineage which respond to even very low doses of LPS. The transcriptional response to LPS is often associated with the activation of NF-κB, which plays an integral role in the immune response [35, 36]. Other tissues such as epithelial cells respond only poorly to an LPS challenge, and proinflammatory cytokines seem to act as the main inducers of chemokine expression [5, 6, 10, 37]. On the other hand, proinflammatory cytokines are, at best, only weakly inducible by chemokines.

CC-chemokines such as MCP-1, RANTES, and MIP-1α/β are inducible by IFN [37–39]. However, contradictory results have been published which show that IFN-γ inhibits the LPS-inducible MCP-1 expression in mouse peritoneal macrophages [40]. The strongest inducer on the transcriptional level of the non-ELR CXC-chemokines IP-10 and MIG has been shown to be IFN-γ [41, 42] via an interferon-stimulated response element (ISRE) as determined for the IP-10 promoter [27, 43, 44], suggesting that both chemokines play an integral role in anti-viral defense after a primary IFN-response. The IFN-γ-responsive element of the Mig promoter as well

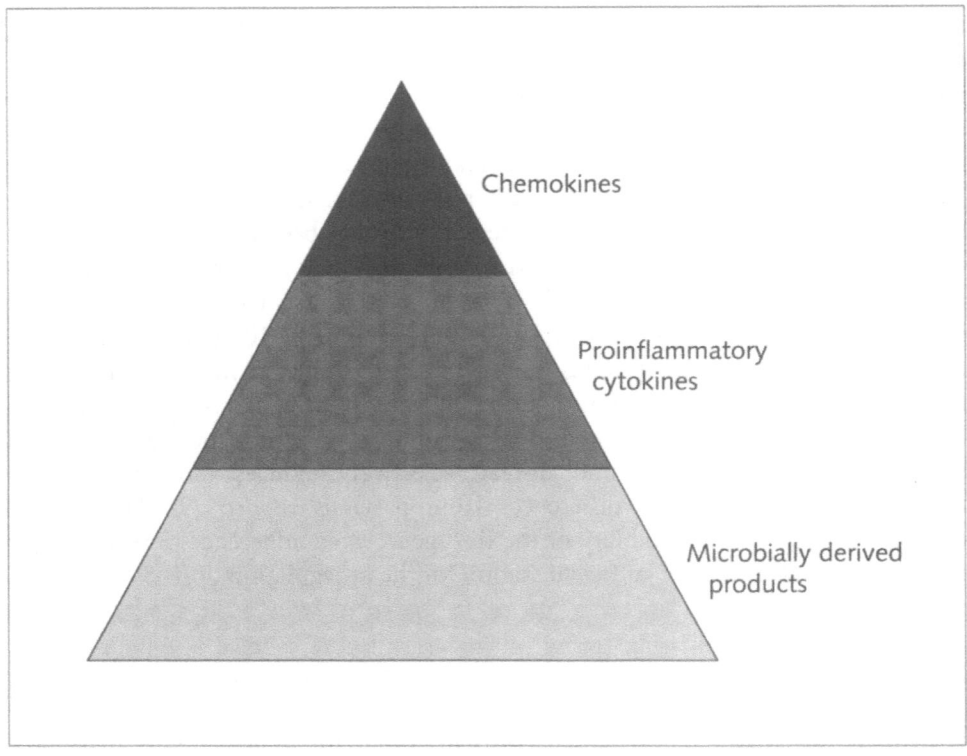

Figure 1
Hierarchy of mediators involved in inflammatory reactions. Microbially-derived products, for example, of bacteria or viruses, can initiate inflammatory reactions by the induction of a wide variety of proinflammatory cytokines in many tissues. Proinflammatory cytokines such as TNF-α and IL-1 are characterized by extremely pleiotropic actions, among them the upregulation of chemokine production. Chemokines have to be considered as secondary mediators responsible for the selective recruitment and fine-tuned activation of distinct effector cell populations. A direct induction of chemokine expression by bacteria or viruses in monocytes and macrophages has also been published. However, the reverse, that chemokines regulate the expression of proinflammatory cytokines is of minor importance.

as the corresponding binding factor are unique and differ from those identified in the IP-10 promoter [45]. The IL-12 induced expression of IP-10 *in vivo* in a mouse tumor model also seems to depend on IFN-γ [46]. LPS, known to be a powerful inducer of other CXC-chemokines in monocytes and macrophages, only inconsistently induces IP-10 in monocytes or neutrophils ([47] and our own unpublished observations). The promoter of the murine IP-10 gene has been shown to contain two distinct NF-κB motifs which are bound by members of the κB sequence binding factors after stimulation with LPS or TNF-α [43, 44]. However, one of them is preferentially bound by the p50/p50 homodimer which functions as a rather suppressive signal [48] and may explain the inconsistent induction of IP-10 by LPS. In contrast, the expression of ELR-CXC-chemokines such as IL-8, GRO, and ENA-78 seems to be downregulated at the transcriptional level by IFN in monocytes and neutrophils [33, 40, 49–51]. The IL-2 stimulated IL-8 expression in human monocytes is inhibited by IFN-γ [52]. The same is true for the LPS-induced IL-8 expression in human granulocytes, which seems to be predominantly downregulated at the transcriptional level [53]. IL-8 suppression by IFN seems to be conferred by factors binding to the NF-κB and NF-IL-6 sites between nucleotides -94 and -71 relative to the start site of transcription [33, 54]. In addition, anti-inflammatory cytokines such as IL-4 and IL-10 have been shown to downregulate IL-8 expression [55–57]. However, tissue specific differences have been noted: In contrast, IL-4 does not inhibit IL-8 expression in fibroblasts, epithelial, and endothelial cells. IFN-γ has been shown to enhance the TNF-induced IL-8 expression in keratinocytes.

With regard to the TH1-/TH2 model of immune regulation, RANTES production has been reported to be inducible by TH1-derived cytokines, while the TH2-derived cytokines, IL-4, IL-10, and IL-13 inhibit its expression [58, 59]. IL-4 treatment decreased the superantigen-induced expression of RANTES, but not of IL-8 in human synoviocytes [60]. IL-10, as an antagonist of IFN-γ-actions, has been shown to suppress the production of IP-10 [47]. Furthermore, IL-4 and IL-10 inhibit MIP-1α and MIP-1β expression by accelerating the decay of chemokine mRNAs [57, 61]. An additional suppressive effect of IL-4 and IL-10 on the LPS- and cytokine-induced transcriptional activation of the MIP-1α gene in human monocytes and alveolar macrophages has been reported [61, 62]. The prototype TH1-cytokine, IFN-γ, is a potent inducer of MCP-1, but not of IL-8, in endothelial cells [63]. The role of TH2-cytokines in the regulation of MCP-1 expression is more complex, in that the typical TH2-associated inhibitory effects are predominantly mediated by IL-4 and IL-13, while IL-10 seems to augment spontaneous MCP-1 expression [64]. On the contrary, IL-4 secretion by the main promoters of a TH2-polarization, CD4+NK1+ T cells, has been shown to induce MCP-1 in spleen cells in a mouse model of listeriosis [65]. In general, the expression of CC- and non-ELR-CXC-chemokines seems to be associated with a TH1-polarized immune response [66], while a TH2-response leads to their suppression (Tab. 1).

Such differences in the inducible expression of functionally related chemokine subsets may explain the appearance of distinct leukocyte populations at sites of inflammation and injury, as we found after infection with influenza virus [22]. IL-8 production in monocytes has been shown to be inhibited by anti-inflammatory drugs such as corticoids. IL-8 suppression by glucocorticoids seems to be conferred by factors binding to the NF-κB and NF-IL-6 sites between nucleotides -94 and -71

Table 1 - *Chemokine expression during TH1/TH2-polarized immune responses*

		TH1-cytokines (e.g. IFN-γ, IL-12)	TH2-cytokines (e.g. IL-4, IL-10, IL-13)	References
ELR-CXC[a]	IL-8	↓	↓ (↔?)	[33, 49–57, 60, 63]
	GRO	↓	ND	[40]
	ENA-78	↓	ND	[51]
nonELR-CXC	IP-10	↑↑	↓	[27, 41–44, 47]
	MIG	↑↑	ND	[42, 45, 95]
CC	MCP-1	↑ (↓?)	↓ (↑?)	[38–40, 63–65]
	MIP-1α/β	↑	↓	[39, 57, 61, 62, 66]
	RANTES	↑	↓	[37, 58–60, 66]

[a] *CXC refers to the first essential cysteine residues of the CXC-branch of chemokines which are interrupted by an intervening amino acid while both cysteines are expressed directly adjacent in the CC-branch. All chemokines with predominantly neutrophil attracting activity express an aminoterminally located ELR-motif. (↑) inducible, (↔) no effect, (↓) suppressed, (ND) not determined.*

relative to the start site of transcription [33, 54]. Generally, glucocorticoids seem to be the most powerful inhibitors of CXC- as well as CC-chemokine expression [37, 67, 68].

Mechanisms of chemokine gene regulation

Despite a clustered genomic localization and a similar genomic structure of members of the same branch, their promoter regions appear to be quite divergent. CC-chemokines map to 17, q11-21 and consist of three exons and two introns while CXC-chemokines are located on chromosome 4, q12-21 and consist of four exons and three introns (already reviewed in [6]). Chemokines appear to be encoded by single copy genes. Important transcription factor binding sites such as those for NF-κB are not consistently found throughout all chemokine promoters despite their inducibility as immediate- or early response genes.

Chemokine gene expression after stimulation with proinflammatory cytokines is at least partly due to transcriptional activation, as shown by nuclear run-off assays and *de novo* synthesis. In addition, cycloheximide enhances the expression of many chemokine genes, most likely by inhibiting the synthesis of short-lived repressor elements (reviewed in [6]). However, in striking contrast to IL-8, the onset of LPS- or cytokine-induced ENA-78 expression in monocytes started after some delay and was completely abrogated in the presence of cycloheximide [67]. This was also found for MCP-1 at least in monocytes, since cycloheximide abolishes LPS- and virus-induced MCP-1 expression, suggesting an indirect induction via newly synthesized protein factors ([38] and our own unpublished observations). A posttranscriptional regulation of chemokine expression has to be anticipated, since most chemokine mRNAs bear AU-rich elements in their 3'-UTR [69, 70] which have been shown to confer mRNA instability in other cytokine mRNAs [71]. An extremely prolonged half-life of IL-8 mRNA has been found at 24 h after stimulation with LPS. This prolonged half-life was higher than it had been after 2 h, suggesting a time-dependent up-regulation of mRNA stability [72].

The promoter region of IL-8 is typical of genes inducible by inflammatory processes. It possesses putative binding sites for several known transcription factors such as NF-κB, NF-IL-6 (C/EBP), AP-1, IRF-1, NF-PMA, an octamer-binding motif, and a GRE [73, 74]. A relatively small region of the human IL-8 gene up to position -94 which includes the NF-κB and NF-IL-6 binding sites as well as the TATA-box was identified to serve as the minimal promoter element responsive to proinflammatory cytokines and PHA [74]. Binding of NF-κB and NF-IL-6 to this region has been demonstrated by gel-shift assays. RelA (p65), but not NFκB1 (p50), seems to be the major component of the κB binding complexes involved in regulation of the IL-8 promoter [75]. A cooperative binding of associated RelA and NF-IL-6 (C/EBP) within this region results in a synergistic transcriptional activation of the IL-8 gene [76–78].

The immediate 5'-flanking regions of the GRO genes are highly homologous and similarly regulated [79–81]. In particular, the minimal promoter element of the GRO-α gene has been mapped between positions -143 and -62 upstream of the transcription start site to which binding of SP1 and SP-3 is necessary for basal promoter activity [82]. In addition, binding of NF-κB and members of the high mobility group of chromosomal non-histone proteins which bind to AT-rich motifs (HMG-I(Y)) is required for transcriptional activation [82]. In the promoter of the murine homolog, MIP-2, an LPS responsive element has been mapped containing a conserved NF-κB consensus motif immediately upstream of the transcription start site [83].

The basic promoter structures of CC-chemokine genes do not essentially differ from the genes of the CXC-subfamily. Potential binding sites for the common transcription factors NF-κB, NF-IL-6 (C/EBPβ), AP-1, and AP-2 have been identified in the immediate upstream regions of the MCP-1 [84], RANTES [85], IP-10 [41, 43, 44], IL-8 [73], GRO [79], ENA-78 [86] and GCP-2 [87] genes. Except for very closely related genes such as the GRO family or the genes encoding ENA-78 and GCP-2, of which the immediate 5' flanking regions include notable stretches of high similarity (>85%), other regions of chemokine promoters have largely diverged.

LPS responsive elements have been mapped at similar positions in the immediate 5'-flanking regions of the murine RANTES and IP-10 genes which resemble AP-1 and ISRE sites while NF-κB binding sites were of minor importance [88]. Among the proteins binding to these motifs after LPS stimulation, c-Jun and CREB, but not other members of the AP-1 family of transcription factors, have been identified by EMSA. The same region of the murine RANTES promoter has been shown to confer transcriptional induction by Newcastle Disease Virus [89]. Again, c-Jun was identified to bind to this virus responsive element and NF-κB was found to be of minor importance. However, instead of CREB, binding of a factor of the high mobility group of chromosomal non-histone proteins (HMG-I(Y)) was demonstrated. This suggests that the basic virus and LPS responsive elements may share extensive sequence homology and that distant enhancer elements may explain the differences in the stimulus-specific gene expression patterns. Members of the C/EBP, NF-κB and c-Ets family of nuclear binding proteins have been shown to bind to a DNAseI-hypersensitive site in the proximal promoter of the murine MIP-1α gene after stimulation with LPS [90]. However, by transient transfection analyses of 5'-deletion constructs of the human MIP-1α promoter, in which highly homologous sites are located at similar positions, we could reproducibly demonstrate that the potential NF-κB like site was not part of the LPS responsive element. A proximal sequence 127 to 51 bp upstream of the transcription start site of the murine MIP-1β gene is bound by members of the ATF/CREB family of transcription factors and serves as an LPS-responsive element [91].

The RANTES promoter region contains four NF-κB sites essentially involved in gene regulation, of which the two distant ones (position -213, and -579 relative to the transcription start site) overlap with an NF-AT binding site and a CD28-responsive element, respectively [92]. The two tandemly arranged κB-like sequences in close proximity of the transcription start site bind not only to Rel family members but also to late expressed non-Rel factors (responsive region: -71 to -53) upregulated 3 to 5 days following activation [93]. In T lymphocytes two distinct expression patterns of the RANTES gene can be distinguished from each other: The immediate early expression in some cell types seems to depend on NF-IL-6/C/EBPβ-binding to sequences from -115 to -91 relative to the transcription start site, while a region from -195 to -144 of the RANTES promoter binds to apparently novel factors which contribute to the late transcriptional upregulation after 3 to 5 days in normal T cells [94]. The region in between seems to be essential for LPS-inducibility [88]. The cooperative induction by IFN-γ and TNF-α of the genes encoding RANTES and Mig is synergistically mediated by two distinct transcription factors: signal transducer and activator of transcription 1 (STAT1), which was essential, and NF-κB [95].

In contrast, no NF-κB site was involved in LPS-inducibility of the genes encoding MIP-1α and MIP-1β. The 5'-flanking regions of both human MIP-1α and MIP-1β genes share common transcription factor binding motifs and are highly homologous over 2 κB, except a repetitive Alu sequence localized in the β-promoter [96]. Both genes seem to be similarly regulated, and the Alu element appears to be unimportant for the regulation of MIP-1β gene expression. In the promoter of the human MIP-1α gene a negative regulatory element, ICK-1, was identified by EMSA and footprinting analyses in Jurkat T cells. This element was bound by low affinity negative and high affinity positive regulatory proteins of which the most important were designated ICK-1A and ICK-1B, respectively [97]. By contrast, this ICK-1 binding site does not confer negative regulation in monocytic U937 cells. An additional binding site, designated MIP-1α nuclear protein (MNP) site, overlaps the ICK-1 element and seems to be crucial for transcriptional initiation of the human MIP-1α gene [98]. This site seems to play an important role in the balanced expression of MIP-1α, in particular after LPS stimulation or viral infection.

Two consensus AP-1 sites have been found in the immediate 5'-flanking region of the human MCP-1 gene which may be responsible for TPA inducibility in endothelial cells [84, 99]. The induction by IL-1 of the human MCP-1 gene is mediated by transcription factors that bind to an NF-κB-like and an AP-1 site located immediately upstream of the transcription start site [100]. The NF-κB-like site located at position -90 binds to the p50/p65 heterodimer of the NF-κB/Rel family in IL-1β-stimulated human endothelial cells. A GC-box in close proximity to the start site of transcription, most likely bound by SP-1, was found to be important in maintaining basal transcriptional activity. A remote NF-κB site more than 2.6 kB upstream was identified to be the essential enhancer element for TNF-, IL-1-, and TPA-inducible MCP-1 expression [101]. NF-IL6, a member of the C/EBP related protein family has been shown to confer LPS-inducible expression of MCP-1 [102]. A seven-nucleotide motif has been identified in the 3'-UTR of the MCP-1 gene as a putative response element for growth factor inducibility [103].

Chemokine receptors

Chemokines bind to G-protein coupled receptors featuring seven transmembrane spanning domains. The general properties and the biology of chemokine receptors has essentially been reviewed in [8, 9]. The size of approximately 350 amino acids and the genomic structure of CC-chemokine receptors (CCRs) as well as CXC-chemokine receptors (CXCRs) appear to be very similar: The ORFs and 3'-UTRs of these receptors are typically encoded by a single large exon, while parts of the 5'-UTR are encoded by small additional exons. This is also true for the fMLPRs which bind to bacterially-derived formyl-peptides (formyl-Met-Leu-Phe; fMLP) and are abundantly expressed on monocytes, neutrophils, and differentiated myeloid cells [104]. Such "classical" chemoattractants do not show any homology or target cell specificity comparable to that of chemokines.

Tissue-specific and activation state dependent expression of chemokine receptors

Most chemokine receptors are tissue-specifically and constitutively expressed by distinct cell types. Two distinct human IL-8 receptors have been cloned which are abundantly expressed in mature neutrophils [105, 106] and are now designated CXCR1 and -2 according to the new conventions for chemokine receptor nomenclature adopted at the Gordon Conference on Chemotactic Cytokines, June 23–28, 1996. Receptor expression increases with advancing differentiation and maturation of the cells [107–109]. G-CSF enhances, and LPS inhibits IL-8R mRNA expression. The stimulatory effect of G-CSF is transcriptional, while LPS utilizes both transcriptional and posttranscriptional mechanisms for IL-8R downregulation. The essential promoter region of both CXCR1 and 2 was mapped to the immediate region upstream of the transcription start site [107, 108]. In both genes this region appeared to be very GC-rich with SP-1 and AP-2 like sites and nonconsensus TATA boxes, a typical feature of constitutively expressed genes. This minimal promoter region was found to confer constitutive expression, inducibility by G-CSF (shown for CXCR2), and was controlled by silencer elements located further upstream. The relevance of 2 NF-κB-like sites >1000 bp upstream of the transcription start site has not yet been demonstrated and the promoter of CXCR1 does not contain NF-κB sites at all. A sequence alignment highlights multiple stretches of striking homology (Fig. 2) shared by both promoters which may represent regulatory sites for tissue-specific expression and/or cytokine-responsive elements. In addition, expression within the T-lineage of both IL-8Rs, CXCR1 and 2, is restricted to NK-like cells. CXCR3, a receptor that specifically binds to IP-10 and Mig, is selectively expressed in IL-2-activated T- and NK-cells [110]. In contrast, CXCR4, which binds to SDF-1 and serves as a major HIV-coreceptor, is constitutively expressed in a variety of leukocytes and other tissues [111, 112].

Of the cloned CCRs, CCR1 [113, 114] has been found to be expressed in monocytes and lymphocytes while CCR2 A and B [115] is predominantly expressed in monocytes. These two transcripts of the CCR2 are generated by alternative splicing and derived from a single gene. The expression of both variants decreases with advancing differentiation of monocytes into macrophages [116]. As determined by murine cell lines, CCR2 seems to be expressed by monocytic cells while, conversely, the expression of CCR1 seems to be more pronounced in macrophage-like cells [117]. CCR2A contains a carboxyl-terminal cytoplasmic retention signal which is responsible for the predominant localization in the cytoplasm while CCR2B traffics efficiently to the cell surface [118]. Such different products derived from a distinct gene have not been described for other chemokine receptors yet. CCR3 is predominantly found on eosinophils [119, 120] and CCR4 on basophils [121]. CCR5 seems to be expressed by PBMCs [112, 122]. A novel CCR, suggested designation CCR6, which specifically binds with high affinity to

```
(1)   CXCR1 (1)  -430   TTgAGTgCCT    -421
      CXCR1 (2)    47   TgCAGcTCCT      56
      CXCR2       -582   TTCAGTTCCT    -573

(2)   CXCR1       228   TGGAGTtAGCAGGTG    242
      CXCR2       303   TGGAGAGAGCAGcTG   -289

(3)   CXCR1      -795   CCAGACTCTGGGagTGGcCTA   -775
      CXCR2      -976   CCAGACTCTGGGctTGGgCTA   -956

(4)   CXCR1      -739   GGTCATTGGcA    -729
      CXCR2      -400   GGTCATTGGgA    -390

(5)   CXCR1      -725   TTGtGCGAAAG    -715
      CXCR2      -386   TTG-GCGAAAG    -377

(6)   CXCR1      -565   AGgAGGAAGG    -556
      CXCR2      -361   AGtAGGAAGG    -352

(7)   CXCR1      -376   C-TGGATTgCCCCC    -364
      CXCR2       193   C-TGGATTTCCCCC     205

(8)   CXCR1      -292   CAGGaaGTTGcAAGC    -278
      CXCR2      -743   CAGGgtGTTGtAAGC    -729

(9)   CXCR1      -102   ACAAGTCtGT    -93
      CXCR2       -68   ACAAGTCcGT    -59

(10)  CXCR1       -75   TGTTCTTCCCC     -65
      CXCR2     -1058   TGTTCTTCCCC   -1048

(11)  CXCR1       -61   TGtAGACATgGGTGG    -47
      CXCR2       299   TGaAGACATcGGTGG    313

(12)  CXCR1       -42   CAGAaGGGAGGTG    -30
      CXCR2      -322   CAGAgGGGAGGTG   -310

(13)  CXCR1        30   AGTCACTCTGAtC     40
      CXCR2      -113   tcTCACTCTGACC   -103

(14)  CXCR1        38   ATCTCTGAC     46
      CXCR2      -887   ATCTCTGAC   -879
```

Figure 2
Alignment of the promoter regions of the human CXCR1 and CXCR2 genes. The sequences
of both promoters were analyzed using the "Gap-" and "Bestfit-" functions of the sequence
analysis software package of the Genetics Computer Group (GCG, Madison, WI). Only the
motifs with at least 80% sequence similarity over at least 10 consecutive nucleotides are
shown. Identical bases are represented by capital letters.

the recently cloned lymphocyte-directed chemokine LARC (liver and activation-regulated chemokine), is selectively expressed on lymphocytes and strongly upregulated by IL-2 [123].

Regulation by cytokines and bacterially-derived molecules

The immediate short-term regulation of chemokine receptors after ligand binding is mediated by means of C-terminal phosphorylation by receptor-specific kinases within seconds. Thereafter, the receptors are internalized within minutes, and finally recycled and reexpressed on the cell surface [124, 125]. In addition, the affinity of the receptors for the ligand is altered after intracellular binding of the G protein. These events lead to desensitization of the receptor response within minutes. However, a long-term regulation of receptor gene expression effective within hours is mediated by cytokines and bacterially-derived molecules.

Only limited data is available concerning the regulation of gene expression of chemokine receptors. CCR1, CCR2, and CCR3 are IL-2 inducible genes that are only minimally expressed on quiescent T cells [126]. This seems to be applicable to all cloned CCRs. However, activation of fully responsive lymphocytes through the TCR/CD3 complex rapidly downregulates receptor expression. IL-2 has also been reported to upregulate CCR2 expression in human NK cells [127]. LPS, and to a lesser extent, IL-1 and TNF-α, have been shown to reduce mRNA expression of the chemokine receptors CCR1, CCR2, and CCR5 [128]. The downregulation by the proinflammatory cytokines IL-1 and TNF-α was most pronounced for CCR2 expression and mediated at the level of gene transcription [129]. Down-regulation of CCR2 expression was also found following differentiation of THP-1 cells into macrophages with PMA or after treatment with IFN-γ [116, 129].

Two distinct research areas, virology and immunology have recently converged in the investigation of the pathogenesis of HIV. The chemokine receptors CXCR4 and CCR5 have been identified as critical HIV co-receptors of virus entry which determine T cell and macrophage-tropism, respectively [130, 131]. Spontaneous CCR5 expression can vary by 20-fold on cells from individuals with homozygously intact alleles for as yet unknown reasons [132]. A strong constitutive expression of CCR5 has been found on previously activated T cells of the memory phenotype (CD45R0$^+$), rendering them highly susceptible for HIV infection [112]. In comparison, CXCR4 expression is higher on naïve, inactivated cells. In addition, CXCR4 expression is rapidly upregulated during PHA-stimulation and priming by IL-2 [112]. Thus, the activation state of T cells and the differential expression patterns of CXCR4 and CCR5 are critical hallmarks not only for lymphocyte migration, but also for HIV susceptibility.

Acknowledgements
We are grateful to L. Perry for providing expert editorial assistance.

References

1   Tanaka Y, Adams DH, Hubscher S, Hirano H, Siebenlist U, Shaw S (1993) T cell adhesion induced by proteoglycan-immobilized cytokine MIP-1β. *Nature* 361: 79–82
2   Springer TA (1994) Traffic signals for lymphocyte recirculation and leukocyte emigration: the multistep paradigm. *Cell* 76: 301–314
3   Imhof BA, Dunon D (1995) Leukocyte migration and adhesion. *Adv Immunol* 58: 345–416
4   Hedrick JA, Zlotnik A (1996) Chemokines and lymphocyte biology. *Curr Opin Immunol* 8: 343–347
5   Oppenheim JJ, Zachariae COC, Mukaida N, Matsushima K (1991) Properties of the novel proinflammatory supergene "intercrine" cytokine family. *Annu Rev Immunol* 9: 617–648
6   Baggiolini M, Dewald B, Moser B (1994) Interleukin-8 and related chemotactic cytokines – CXC and CC chemokines. *Adv Immunol* 55: 97–179
7   Schall TJ, Bacon KB (1994) Chemokines, leukocyte trafficking, and inflammation. *Curr Opin Immunol* 6: 865–873
8   Kelvin DJ, Michiel DF, Johnston JA, Lloyd AR, Sprenger H, Oppenheim JJ, Wang J-M (1993) Chemokines and serpentines: the molecular biology of chemokine receptors. *J Leukoc Biol* 54: 604–612
9   Murphy PM (1994) The molecular biology of leukocyte chemoattractant receptors. *Annu Rev Immunol* 12: 593–633
10   Baggiolini M, Dewald B, Moser B (1997) Human chemokines: An update. *Annu Rev Immunol* 15: 675–705
11   Fahey TJ, Sherry B, Tracey KJ, van Deventer S, Jones WG, Minei JP, Morgello S, Shires GT, Cerami A (1990) Cytokine production in a model of wound healing: The appearance of MIP-1, MIP-2, cachectin TNF and IL-1. *Cytokine* 2: 92–99
12   Iida N, Grotendorst GR (1990) Cloning and sequencing of a new gro transcript from activated human monocytes: Expression in leukocytes and wound tissue. *Mol Cell Biol* 10: 5596–5599
13   Koch AE, Polverini PJ, Kunkel SL, Harlow LA, DiPietro LA, Elner VM, Elner SG, Strieter RM (1992) Interleukin-8 as a macrophage-derived mediator of angiogenesis. *Science* 258: 1798–1801
14   Shibata Y, Nakamura H, Kato S, Tomoike H (1996) Cellular detachment and deformation induce IL-8 gene expression in human bronchial epithelial cells. *J Immunol* 156: 772–777
15   Angiolillo AL, Sgadari C, Taub DD, Liao F, Farber JM, Maheshwari S, Kleinman HK,

Reaman GH, Tosato G (1995) Human interferon-inducible protein 10 is a potent inhibitor of angiogenesis *in vivo*. *J Exp Med* 182: 155–162

16   Arenberg DA, Kunkel SL, Polverini PJ, Morris SB, Burdick MD, Glass MC, Taub DD, Iannettoni MD, Whyte RI, Strieter RM (1996) Interferon-γ-inducible protein 10 (IP-10) is an angiostatic factor that inhibits human non-small cell lung cancer (NSCLC) tumorigenesis and spontaneous metastases. *J Exp Med* 184: 981–992

17   Luster AD, Greenberg SM, Leder P (1995) The IP-10 chemokine binds to a specific cell surface heparan sulfate site shared with platelet factor 4 and inhibits endothelial cell proliferation. *J Exp Med* 182: 219–231

18   Petzelbauer P, Watson CA, Pfau SE, Pober JS (1995) IL-8 and angiogenesis: evidence that human endothelial cells lack receptors and do not respond to IL-8 *in vitro*. *Cytokine* 7: 267–272

19   Schönbeck U, Brandt E, Petersen F, Flad H-D, Loppnow H (1995) IL-8 specifically binds to endothelial but not to smooth muscle cells. *J Immunol* 154: 2375–2383

20   Cao Y, Chen C, Weatherbee JA, Tsang M, Folkman J (1995) Gro-β, a CXC-chemokine, is an angiogenesis inhibitor that suppresses the growth of Lewis lung carcinoma in mice. *J Exp Med* 182: 2069–2077

21   Carp H (1982) Mitochondrial N-formylmethionyl proteins as chemoattractants for neutrophils. *J Exp Med* 155: 264–275

22   Sprenger H, Meyer RG, Kaufmann A, Bubfeld D, Rischkowsky E, Gemsa D (1996) Selective induction of monocyte and not neutrophil-attracting chemokines after influenza A virus infection. *J Exp Med* 184: 1191–1196

23   Cook DN, Beck MA, Coffman TM, Kirby SL, Sheridan JF, Pragnell IB, Smithies O (1995) Requirement of MIP-1α for an inflammatory response to viral infection. *Science* 269: 1583–1585

24   Cocchi F, DeVico AL, Garzino-Demo A, Arya SK, Gallo RC, Lusso P (1995) Identification of RANTES, MIP-1α, and MIP-1β as the major HIV-suppressive factors produced by CD8+ T cells. *Science* 270: 1811–1815

25   van Damme J, Proost P, Put W, Arens S, Lenaerts J-P, Conings R, Opdenakker G, Heremans H, Billiau A (1994) Induction of monocyte chemotactic proteins MCP-1 and MCP-2 in human fibroblasts and leukocytes by cytokines and cytokine inducers. *J Immunol* 152: 5495–5502

26   Vanguri P, Farber JM (1994) IFN and virus-inducible expression of an immediate early gene, crg-2/IP-10, and a delayed gene, I-Aa, in astrocytes and microglia. *J Immunol* 152: 1411–1418

27   Nazar AS, Cheng G, Shin HS, Brothers PN, Dhib-Jalbut S, Shin ML, Vanguri P (1997) Induction of IP-10 chemokine promoter by measles virus: comparison with interferon-γ shows the use of the same response element but with differential DNA-protein binding profiles. *J Neuroimmunol* 77: 116–127

28   van Damme J, Decock B, Conings R, Lenaerts J-P, Opdenakker G, Billiau A (1989) The chemotactic activity for granulocytes produced by virally infected fibroblasts is identical to monocyte-derived interleukin 8. *Eur J Immunol* 19: 1189–1194

29 Choi AMK, Jacoby DB (1992) Influenza virus A infection induces interleukin-8 gene expression in human airway epithelial cells. *FEBS Lett* 309: 327–329

30 Becker S, Quay J, Soukoup J (1991) Cytokine (tumor necrosis factor, IL-6, and IL-8) production by respiratory syncytial virus-infected human alveolar macrophages. *J Immunol* 147: 4307–4312

31 Subauste MC, Jacoby DB, Richards SM, Proud D (1995) Infection of a human respiratory epithelial cell line with rhinovirus. Induction of cytokine release and modulation of susceptibility to infection by cytokine exposure. *J Clin Invest* 96: 549–557

32 Panuska JR, Merolla R, Rebert NA, Hoffmann SP, Tsivitse P, Cirino NM, Silverman RH, Rankin JA (1995) Respiratory syncytial virus induces interleukin-10 by human alveolar macrophages. Suppression of early cytokine production and implications for incomplete immunity. *J Clin Invest* 96: 2445–2453

33 Oliveira IC, Mukaida N, Matsushima K, Vilcek J (1994) Transcriptional inhibition of the interleukin-8 gene by interferon is mediated by the NF-κB site. *Mol Cell Biol* 14: 5300–5308

34 Kasahara K, Strieter RM, Chensue SW, Standiford TJ, Kunkel SL (1991) Mononuclear cell adherence induces neutrophil chemotactic factor/interleukin-8 gene expression. *J Leukoc Biol* 50: 287–295

35 Bäuerle PA, Henkel T (1994) Function and activation of NF-κB in the immune system. *Annu Rev Immunol* 12: 141–179

36 Vincenti MP, Burrell TA, Taffet SM (1992) Regulation of NF-kappa B activity in murine macrophages: Effect of bacterial lipopolysaccharide and phorbol ester. *J Cell Physiol* 150: 204–213

37 Stellato S, Beck LA, Gorgone GA, Proud D, Schall TJ, Ono SJ, Lichtenstein LM, Schleimer RP (1995) Expression of the chemokine RANTES by a human bronchial epithelial cell line. Modulation by cytokines and glucocorticoids. *J Immunol* 155: 410–418

38 Colotta F, Borré A, Wang J-M, Tattanelli M, Maddalena F, Polentarutti N, Peri G, Mantovani A (1992) Expression of a monocyte chemotactic cytokine by human mononuclear phagocytes. *J Immunol* 148: 760–765

39 Martin CA, Dorf ME (1991) Differential regulation of interleukin-6, macrophage inflammatory protein-1, and JE/MCP-1 cytokine expression in macrophage cell lines. *Cell Immunol* 135: 245–258

40 Ohmori Y, Hamilton TA (1994) IFN-γ selectively inhibits lipopolysaccharide-inducible JE/monocytes chemoattractant protein-1 and KC/GRO/melanoma growth-stimulating activity gene expression in mouse peritoneal macrophages. *J Immunol* 153: 2204–2212

41 Luster AD, Ravetch JV (1987) Genomic characterization of a γ-interferon-inducible gene (IP-10) and identification of an interferon-inducible hypersensitive site. *Mol Cell Biol* 7: 3723–3731

42 Farber JM (1997) Mig and IP-10: CXC chemokines that target lymphocytes. *J Leukoc Biol* 61: 246–257

43 Ohmori Y, Hamilton TA (1993) Cooperative interaction between interferon (IFN) stim-

ulus response element and κB sequence motifs controls IFNγ- and lipopolysaccharide-stimulated transcription from the murine IP-10 promoter. *J Biol Chem* 268: 6677–6688

44 Ohmori Y, Hamilton TA (1995) The interferon-stimulated response element and a κB site mediate synergistic induction of murine IP-10 gene transcription by IFN-γ and TNF-α. *J Immunol* 154: 5235–5244

45 Wong P, Severns CW, Guyer NB, Wright TM (1994) A unique palindromic element mediates gamma interferon induction of mig gene expression. *Mol Cell Biol* 14: 914–922

46 Tannenbaum CS, Wicker N, Armstrong D, Tubbs R, Finke J, Bukowski RM, Hamilton TA (1996) Cytokine and chemokine expression in tumors of mice receiving systemic therapy with IL-12. *J Immunol* 156: 693–699

47 Cassatella MA, Gasperini S, Calzetti F, Bertagnin A, Luster AD, MacDonald PP (1997) Regulated production of the interferon-γ-inducible protein-10 (IP-10) chemokine by human neutrophils. *Eur J Immunol* 27: 111–115

48 Ohmori Y, Tebo J, Nedospasov S, Hamilton TA (1994) κB binding activity in a murine macrophage-like cell line. *J Biol Chem* 269: 17684-17690

49 Cassatella MA, Guasparri I, Ceska M, Bazzoni F, Rossi F (1993) Interferon-γ inhibits interleukin-8 production by human polymorphonuclear leukocytes. *Immunology* 78: 177–184

50 Oliveira IC, Sciavolino PJ, Lee TH, Vilcek J (1992) Downregulation of interleukin 8 gene expression in human fibroblasts: Unique mechanism of transcriptional inhibition by interferon. *Proc Natl Acad Sci USA* 89: 9049–9053

51 Schnyder-Candrian S, Strieter RM, Kunkel SL, Walz A (1995) Interferon-α and interferon-γ down-regulate the production of interleukin-8 and ENA-78 in human monocytes. *J Leukoc Biol* 57: 929–935

52 Gusella GL, Musso T, Bosco MC, Espinoza-Delgado I, Matsushima K, Varesio L (1993) IL-2 up-regulates but IFN-γ suppresses IL-8 expression in human monocytes. *J Immunol* 151: 2725–2732

53 Cassatella MA, Gasperini S, Calzetti F, McDonald PP, Trinchieri G (1995) Lipopolysaccharide-induced interleukin-8 gene expression in human granulocytes: transcriptional inhibition by interferon-gamma. *Biochem J* 310: 751–755

54 Mukaida N, Okamoto S, Ishikawa Y, Matsushima K (1994) Molecular mechanism of interleukin-8 gene expression. *J Leukoc Biol* 56: 554–558

55 Standiford TJ, Strieter RM, Chensue SW, Westwick J, Kasahara K, Kunkel SL (1990) IL-4 inhibits the expression of IL-8 from stimulated human monocytes. *J Immunol* 145: 1435–1439

56 De Waal Malefyt R, Abrams J, Bennett B, Figdor CG, de Vries JE (1991) Interleukin 10 (IL-10) inhibits cytokine synthesis by human monocytes: An autoregulatory role of IL-10 produced by monocytes. *J Exp Med* 174: 1209–1220

57 Kasama T, Strieter RM, Lukacs NW, Burdick MD, Kunkel SL (1994) Regulation of neutrophil-derived chemokine expression by IL-10. *J Immunol* 152: 3559–3569

58 John M, Hirst SJ, Jose PJ, Robichaud A, Berkman N, Witt C, Twort CH, Barnes PJ,

Chung KF (1997) Human airway smooth muscle cells express and release RANTES in response to T helper 1 cytokines: regulation by T helper 2 cytokines and corticosteroids. *J Immunol* 158: 1841–1847

59 Marfaing-Koka A, Devergne O, Gorgone G, Portier A, Schall TJ, Galanaud P, Emilie D (1995) Regulation of the production of the RANTES chemokine by endothelial cells. Synergistic induction by IFN-γ plus TNF-α and inhibition by IL-4 and IL-13. *J Immunol* 154: 1870–1878

60 Mehindate K, al-Daccak R, Schall TJ, Mourad W (1994) Induction of chemokine gene expression by major histocompatibility complex class II ligands in human fibroblast-like synoviocytes. Differential regulation by interleukin-4 and dexamethasone. *J Biol Chem* 269: 32063–32069

61 Standiford TJ, Kunkel SL, Liebler JM, Burdick MD, Gilbert AR, Strieter RM (1993) Gene expression of macrophage inflammatory protein-1α from human blood monocytes and alveolar macrophages is inhibited by interleukin-4. *Am J Respir Cell Mol Biol* 9: 192–198

62 Berkman N, John M, Roesems G, Jose PJ, Barnes PJ, Chung KF (1995) Inhibition of macrophage inflammatory protein-1α expression by IL-10. Differential sensitivities in human blood monocytes and alveolar macrophages. *J Immunol* 155: 4412–4418

63 Brown Z, Gerritsen ME, Carley WW, Strieter RM, Kunkel SL, Westwick J (1994) Chemokine gene expression and secretion by cytokine-activated human microvascular endothelial cells. Differential regulation of monocyte chemoattractant protein-1 and interleukin-8 in response to interferon-γ. *Am J Pathol* 145: 913–921

64 Yano S, Yanagawa H, Nishioka Y, Mukaida N, Matsushima K, Sone S (1996) T helper 2 cytokines differently regulate monocyte chemoattractant protein-1 production by human peripheral blood monocytes and alveolar macrophages. *J Immunol* 157: 2660– 2665

65 Flesch IE, Wandersee A, Kaufmann SH (1997) IL-4 secretion by CD4+ NK1+ T cells induces monocyte chemoattractant protein-1 in early listeriosis. *J Immunol* 159: 7-10

66 Schrum S, Probst P, Fleischer B, Zipfel PF (1996) Synthesis of the CC-chemokines MIP-1α, MIP-1β, and RANTES is associated with a type 1 immune response. *J Immunol* 157: 3598–3604

67 Schnyder-Candrian S, Walz A (1997) Neutrophil-activating protein ENA-78 and IL-8 exhibit different patterns of expression in lipopolysaccharide- and cytokine-stimulated human monocytes. *J Immunol* 158: 3888–3894

68 Smith JB, Herschman HR (1995) Glucocorticoid-attenuated response genes encode intercellular mediators, including a new CXC chemokine. *J Biol Chem* 270: 16756–16765

69 Stoeckle MY (1991) Post-transcriptional regulation of groα, β, γ, and IL-8 mRNAs by IL-1β. *Nucleic Acids Res* 19: 917–920

70 Stoeckle MY (1992) Removal of a 3' non-coding sequence is an initial step in degradation of groa mRNA and is regulated by interleukin-1. *Nucleic Acids Res* 20: 1123–1127

71 Shaw G, Kamen R (1986) A conserved AU sequence from the 3' untranslated region of GM-CSF mRNA mediates selective mRNA degradation. *Cell* 46: 659–667

72 Villarete LH, Remick DG (1996) Transcriptional and post-transcriptional regulation of interleukin-8. *Am J Pathol* 149: 1685–1693

73 Mukaida N, Shiroo M, Matsushima K (1989) Genomic structure of the human monocyte-derived neutrophil chemotactic factor IL-8. *J Immunol* 143: 1366–1371

74 Mukaida N, Mahé Y, Matsushima K (1990) Cooperative interaction of nuclear factor-kappaB- and cis-regulatory enhancer binding protein-like factor binding elements in activating the interleukin-8 gene by pro-inflammatory cytokines. *J Biol Chem* 265: 21128–21133

75 Kunsch C, Rosen CA (1993) NF-kappa B subunit-specific regulation of the interleukin-8 promoter. Mol Cell Biol 13: 6137–6146

76 Kunsch C, Lang RK, Rosen CA, Shannon MF (1994) Synergistic transcriptional activation of the IL-8 gene by NF-kappa B p65 (RelA) and NF-IL-6. *J Immunol* 153: 153–164

77 Matsusaka T, Fujikawa K, Nishio Y, Mukaida N, Matsushima K, Kishimoto T, Akira S (1993) Transcription factors NF-IL6 and NF-kappa B synergistically activate transcription of the inflammatory cytokines, interleukin 6 and interleukin 8. *Proc Natl Acad Sci USA* 90: 10193–10197

78 Stein B, Baldwin Jr AS (1993) Distinct mechanisms for regulation of the interleukin-8 gene involve synergism and cooperativity between C/EBP and NF-kappa B. *Mol Cell Biol* 13: 7191–7198

79 Baker NE, Kucera G, Richmond A (1990) Nucleotide sequence of the human melanoma growth stimulatory activity (MGSA) gene. *Nucleic Acids Res* 18: 6453

80 Anisowicz A, Messineo M, Lee SW, Sager R (1991) An NF-κB-like transcription factor mediates IL-1/TNF-α induction of *gro* in human fibroblasts. *J Immunol* 147: 520–527

81 Ohmori Y, Fukumoto S, Hamilton TA (1995) Two structurally distinct κB sequence motifs cooperatively control LPS-induced KC gene transcription in mouse macrophages. *J Immunol* 155: 3593–3600

82 Wood LD, Farmer AA, Richmond A (1995) HMGI(Y) and Sp1 in addition to NF-kappa B regulate transcription of the MGSA/GRO alpha gene. *Nucleic Acids Res* 23: 4210–4219

83 Widmer U, Manogue KR, Cerami A, Sherry B (1993) Genomic cloning and promoter analysis of macrophage inflammatory protein (MIP)-2, MIP-1α, and MIP-1β, members of the chemokine superfamily of proinflammatory cytokines. *J Immunol* 150: 4996–5012

84 Shyy Y-J, Li Y-S, Kolattukudy PE (1990) Structure of human monocyte chemotactic protein gene and its regulation by TPA. *Biochem Biophys Res Commun* 169: 346–351

85 Nelson PJ, Kim HT, Manning WC, Goralski TJ, Krensky AM (1993) Genomic organization and transcriptional regulation of the RANTES chemokine gene. *J Immunol* 151: 2601–2612

86 Chang MS, McNinch J, Basu R, Simonet S (1994) Cloning and characterization of the human neutrophil-activating peptide (ENA-78) gene. *J Biol Chem* 269: 25277–25282

87 Rovai LE, Herschman HR, Smith JB (1997) Cloning and characterization of the human granulocyte chemotactic protein-2 gene. *J Immunol* 158: 5257–5266

88 Shin HS, Drysdale B-E, Shin ML, Noble PW, Fisher SN, Paznekas WA (1994) Definition of a lipopolysaccharide-responsive element in the 5'-flanking regions of muRANTES and *crg*-2. *Mol Cell Biol* 14: 2914–2925

89 Lokuta MA, Maher J, Noe KH, Pitha PM, Shin ML, Shin HS (1996) Mechanisms of murine RANTES chemokine gene induction by Newcastle disease virus. *J Biol Chem* 271: 13731–13738

90 Grove M, Plumb M (1993) C/EBP, NF-κB, and c-ETS family members and transcriptional regulation of the cell-specific and inducible macrophage inflammatory protein 1α immediate-early gene. *Mol Cell Biol* 13: 5276–5289

91 Proffitt J, Crabtree G, Grove M, Daubersies P, Bailleul B, Wright E, Plumb M (1995) An ATF/CREB-binding site is essential for cell-specific and inducible transcription of the murine MIP-1β cytokine gene. *Gene* 152: 173–179

92 Moriuchi H, Moriuchi M, Fauci AS (1997) Nuclear factor-kappa B potently up-regulates the promoter activity of RANTES, a chemokine that blocks HIV infection. *J Immunol* 158: 3483–3491

93 Nelson PJ, Ortiz BD, Pattison JM, Krensky AM (1996) Identification of a novel regulatory region critical for expression of the RANTES chemokine in activated T lymphocytes. *J Immunol* 157: 1139–1148

94 Ortiz BD, Krensky AM, Nelson PJ (1996) Kinetics of transcription factors regulating the RANTES chemokine gene reveal a developmental switch in nuclear events during T-lymphocyte maturation. *Mol Cell Biol* 16: 202–210

95 Ohmori Y, Schreiber RD, Hamilton TA (1997) Synergy between interferon-γ and tumor necrosis factor-α in transcriptional activation is mediated by cooperation between signal transducer and activator of transcription 1 and nuclear factor kappaB. *J Biol Chem* 272: 14899–14907

96 Nakao M, Nomiyama H, Shimada K (1990) Structures of human genes coding for cytokine LD78 and their expression. *Mol Cell Biol* 10: 3646–3658

97 Nomiyama H, Hieshima K, Hirokawa K, Hattori T, Takatsuki K, Miura R (1993) Characterization of cytokine LD78 gene promoters: Positive and negative transcriptional factors bind to a negative regulatory element common to LD78, interleukin-3, and granulocyte-macrophage colony-stimulating factor gene promoters. *Mol Cell Biol* 13: 2787–2801

98 Ritter LM, Bryans M, Abdo O, Sharma V, Wilkie NM (1995) MIP-1α nuclear protein (MNP), a novel transcription factor expressed in hematopoietic cells that is crucial for transcription of the human MIP-1α gene. *Mol Cell Biol* 15: 3110–3118

99 Shyy Y-J, Li Y-S, Kolattukudy PE (1993) Activation of MCP-1 gene expression is mediated through multiple signaling pathways. *Biochem Biophys Res Commun* 192: 693–699

100 Martin T, Cardarelli PM, Parry GC, Felts KA, Cobb RR (1997) Cytokine induction of monocyte chemoattractant protein-1 gene expression in human endothelial cells depends on the cooperative action of NF-κB and AP-1. *Eur J Immunol* 27: 1091–1097

101 Ueda A, Okuda K, Ohno S, Shirai A, Igarashi T, Matsunaga K, Fukushima J, Kawamo-

to S, Ishigatsubo Y, Okubo T (1994) NF-κB and Sp1 regulate transcription of the human monocyte chemoattractant protein-1 gene. *J Immunol* 153: 2052–2063

102 Bretz JD, Williams SC, Baer M, Johnson PF, Schwartz RC (1994) C/EBP-related protein 2 confers lipopolysaccharide-inducible expression of interleukin 6 and monocyte chemoattractant protein 1 to a lymphoblastic cell line. *Proc Natl Acad Sci USA* 91: 7306–7310

103 Freter RR, Irminger J-C, Porter JA, Jones SD, Stiles CD (1992) A novel 7-nucleotide motif located in 3' untranslated sequences of the immediate-early gene set mediates platelet-derived growth factor induction of the JE gene. *Mol Cell Biol* 12: 5288–5300

104 Murphy PM, Tiffany HL, McDermott D, Ahuja SK (1993) Sequence and organization of the human N-formyl peptide receptor-encoding gene. *Gene* 133: 285–290

105 Murphy PM, Tiffany HL (1991) Cloning of complementary DNA encoding a functional interleukin-8 receptor. *Science* 253: 1280–1283

106 Lee J, Horuk R, Rice GC (1992) Characterization of two high affinity human interleukin-8 receptors. *J Biol Chem* 267: 16283–16287

107 Sprenger H, Lloyd AR, Lautens LL, Bonner TI, Kelvin DJ (1994) Structure, genomic organization, and expression of the human interleukin-8 receptor B gene. *J Biol Chem* 269: 11065–11072

108 Sprenger H, Lloyd AR, Meyer RG, Johnston JA, Kelvin DJ (1994) Genomic structure, characterization, and identification of the promoter of the human IL-8 receptor A gene. *J Immunol* 153: 2524–2532

109 Lloyd AR, Biragyn A, Johnston JA, Taub DD, Xu L, Michiel D, Sprenger H, Oppenheim JJ, Kelvin DJ (1995) Granulocyte-colony stimulating factor and lipopolysaccharide regulate the expression of interleukin 8 receptors on polymorphonuclear leukocytes. *J Biol Chem* 270: 28188–28192

110 Loetscher M, Gerber B, Loetscher P, Jones SA, Piali L, Clark-Lewis I, Baggiolini M, Moser B (1996) Chemokine receptor specific for IP-10 and Mig: structure, function, and expression in activated T-lymphocytes. *J Exp Med* 184: 963–969

111 Loetscher M, Geiser T, O'Reilly T, Zwahlen R, Baggiolini M, Moser B (1994) Cloning of a human seven-transmembrane domain receptor, LESTR, that is highly expressed in leukocytes. *J Biol Chem* 269: 232–237

112 Bleul CC, Wu L, Hoxie JA, Springer TA, Mackay CR (1997) The HIV coreceptors CXCR4 and CCR5 are differentially expressed and regulated on human T lymphocytes. *Proc Natl Acad Sci USA* 94: 1925–1930

113 Gao J-L, Kuhns DB, Tiffany HL, McDermott D, Li X, Francke U, Murphy PM (1993) Structure and functional expression of the human macrophage inflammatory protein 1α/RANTES receptor. *J Exp Med* 177: 1421–1427

114 Neote K, DiGregorio D, Mak JY, Horuk R, Schall TJ (1993) Molecular cloning, functional expression, and signalling characteristics of a C-C chemokine receptor. *Cell* 72: 415–425

115 Charo IF, Myers SJ, Herman A, Franci C, Connolly AJ, Coughlin SR (1994) Molecular cloning and functional expression of two monocyte chemoattractant protein 1 receptors

reveals alternative splicing of the carboxyl-terminal tails. *Proc Natl Acad Sci USA* 91: 2752–2756

116 Denholm EM, Stankus GP (1995) Changes in the expression of MCP-1 receptors on monocytic THP-1 cells following differentiation to macrophages with phorbol myristate acetate. *Cytokine* 7: 436–440

117 Boring L, Gosling J, Monteclaro FS, Lusis AJ, Tsou C-L, Charo IF (1996) Molecular cloning and functional expression of murine JE (monocyte chemoattractant protein 1) and murine macrophage inflammatory protein 1α receptors. *J Biol Chem* 271: 7551–7558

118 Wong LM, Myers SJ, Tsou C-L, Gosling J, Arai H, Charo IF (1997) Organization and differential expression of the human monocyte chemoattractant protein 1 receptor gene. Evidence for the role of the carboxyl-terminal tail in receptor trafficking. *J Biol Chem* 272: 1038–1045

119 Daugherty BL, Siciliano SJ, DeMarino JA, Malkowitz L, Sirotina A, Springer MS (1996) Cloning, expression, and characterization of the human eosinophil eotaxin receptor. *J Exp Med* 183: 2349–2354

120 Ponath PD, Qin S, Post TW, Wang J, Wu L, Gerard NP, Newman W, Gerard C, Mackay CR (1996) Molecular cloning and characterization of a human eotaxin receptor expressed selectively on eosinophils. *J Exp Med* 183: 2437–2448

121 Power CA, Meyer A, Nemeth K, Bacon KB, Hoogewerf AJ, Proudfoot AEI, Wells TNC (1995) Molecular cloning and functional expression of a novel CC chemokine receptor cDNA from a human basophilic cell line. *J Biol Chem* 270: 19495–19500

122 Samson M, Labbé O, Mollereau C, Vassart G, Parmentier M (1996) Molecular cloning and functional expression of a new human CC-chemokine receptor gene. *Biochemistry* 35: 3362–3367

123 Baba M, Imai T, Nishimura M, Kakizaki M, Takagi S, Hieshima K, Nomiyama H, Yoshie O (1997) Identification of CCR6, the specific receptor for a novel lymphocyte-directed CC chemokine LARC. *J Biol Chem* 272: 14893–14898

124 Chuntharapai A, Kim KJ (1995) Regulation of the expression of IL-8 receptor A/B by IL-8: possible functions of each receptor. *J Immunol* 155: 2587–2594

125 Franci C, Gosling J, Tsou C-L, Coughlin SR, Charo IF (1996) Phosphorylation by a G protein-coupled kinase inhibits signaling and promotes internalization of the monocyte chemoattractant protein-1 receptor. Critical role of carboxyl-tail serines/threonines in receptor function. *J Immunol* 157: 5606–5612

126 Loetscher P, Seitz M, Baggiolini M, Moser B (1996) Interleukin-2 regulates CC chemokine receptor expression and chemotactic responsiveness in T lymphocytes. *J Exp Med* 184: 569–577

127 Polentarutti N, Allavena P, Bianchi G, Giardina G, Basile A, Sozzani S, Mantovani A, Introna M (1997) IL-2-regulated expression of the monocyte chemotactic protein-1 receptor (CCR2) in human NK cells: characterization of a predominant 3.4-kilobase transcript containing CCR2B and CCR2A sequences. *J Immunol* 158: 2689–2694

128 Sica A, Saccani A, Borsatti A, Power CA, Wells TNC, Luini W, Polentarutti N, Sozzani

S, Mantovani A (1997) Bacterial lipopolysaccharide rapidly inhibits expression of C-C chemokine receptors in human monocytes. *J Exp Med* 185: 969–974

129 Tangirala RK, Murao K, Quehenberger O (1997) Regulation of expression of the human monocyte chemotactic protein-1 receptor (hCCR2) by cytokines. *J Biol Chem* 272: 8050–8056

130 Moore JP, Koup RA (1996) Chemoattractants attract HIV researchers. *J Exp Med* 184: 311–313

131 Bates P (1996) Chemokine receptors and HIV: an attractive pair? *Cell* 86: 1–3

132 Wu L, Paxton WA, Kassam N, Ruffing N, Rottman JB, Sullivan N, Choe H, Sodroski J, Newman W, Koup RA, et al (1997) CCR5 levels and expression pattern correlate with infectability by macrophage-tropic HIV-1, *in vitro*. *J Exp Med* 185: 1681–1691

Chemokines and T lymphocytes

Tan Jinquan[1] and Kristian Thestrup-Pedersen[2]

[1]Department of Immunology, Anhui Medical University, 69 Meishan Road, Hefai 230032, Anhui Province, People's Republic of China
[2]Department of Dermatology, Marselisborg Hospital, University of Aarhus, DK-8000 Aarhus C, Denmark

Introduction

Cellular migration, known as chemotaxis, is a phenomenon that has been studied over the past century. Its relevance in biology was observed by Metchnikoff, who was the first to clearly demonstrate how primary defense mechanisms relied on the migration of inflammatory cells to areas of injury. Later, the focus was on the ability of bacterial products to attract neutrophil granulocytes – the forerunners or "the anti-terrorist corps" in the body's defense against tissue injury or bacterial penetration. Thus, it has been calculated that a neutrophil granulocyte can move 70 times faster than a T lymphocyte. This means that in the days before cell separation became applicable, the cells one saw when studying "cellular migration" were the neutrophil granulocytes. And this was the type of inflammatory response that was observed in all bacterial infections, except a few such as mycobacterial infections.

Several developments with respect to the immune system have allowed for significant improvements in our understanding of chemotaxis. Firstly, we know today that our defense systems are comprised of many important cell types: The phagocytic system (granulocytes and monocytes together with fixed monocytes in tissues, i.e. macrophages), the antigen-presenting system of dendritic cells, and the lymphocytes which are highly specialized cells with many subgroups having different functions. Secondly, we are today able to separate and purify each subgroup of cells and study their behavior with respect to "chemotaxis." This fact is the most important reason why T lymphocyte migration has not been studied until the last two decades.

T lymphocyte migration

Even today there is uncertainty about T lymphocyte migration. In 1989, it was published that IL-8, a CXC chemokine, was chemotactic for human T lymphocytes [1]. However, in 1993, from the same laboratory and in the same journal (*Science*), it was published that IL-8 was not T lymphocyte chemotactic [2].

This fact concerning publications with quite different observations on chemotaxis of T lymphocytes underlines a very important issue when discussing T lymphocytes and chemokines, and these are the technical aspects of how one measures T lymphocyte migration. It applies not only to the performance of the *in vitro* chemotaxis itself, but also to the separation of cells, the time between separation and how cells are handled before being subjected to the chemotaxis assay. It is therefore necessary in this review to first discuss some technical aspects of measuring T lymphocyte migration.

The technical aspects of measuring T lymphocyte migration

Cell separation

The first important issue is the purification process. When isolating mononuclear cells from peripheral blood on Isopaque-Ficoll (1.077 density), one gets a cell mixture where T lymphocytes may form 50–70% of content, B lymphocytes 5–15% and monocytes from 15–45% of the cells. It is very important to remove monocytes, because they have a higher migratory capacity. T cell separation can be done using the old E-rosette technique, where only CD2+ cells will form rosettes. The authors recommend using a suitable donor sheep, and to continue using this donor in order to achieve good reproducibility.

Previously, a cheap and efficient way of T cell purification was the nylon wool method. However, approximately half of the lymphocytes are lost and it is likely that those being most adhesive will disappear. Today, many laboratories use plastic adherence, i.e. 1–2 h incubation of the mononuclear cell population in medium in a plastic flask following isolation of the non-adherent cells, which will be mostly T lymphocytes. This step will remove almost all monocytes (which can then be isolated for other purposes) and also many B cells. Again, the most adhesive T lymphocytes are likely to disappear.

The best separation procedure is the DynaBead technique, where both positive or negative selection can be done – not only of CD3+ T lymphocytes, but also of subsets of T lymphocytes. (The only "side-effects" will be budgetary.)

The microwell technique

One can measure cell migration using either the old Boyden chamber system, which demands large volumes of chemokines and cells, or the Neuroprobe microwell system, which is probably most used today. Both techniques are in principle very simple, but in practice difficult to handle. It is important to realize one thing: Normally one counts the number of cells that have reached the lower chamber in the Boy-

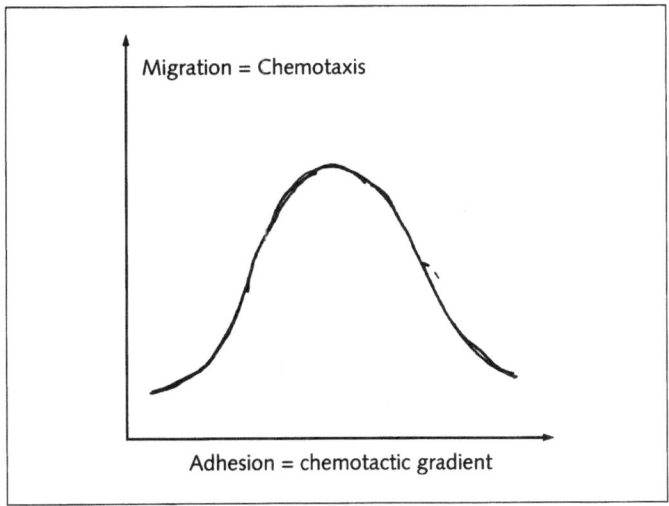

Figure 1
The drawing illustrates how "migration" – or chemotaxis – relates to "adhesion" – or a chemotactic gradient

den system (*migration and drop-down*), whereas the Neuroprobe system measures the amount of cells on the lower part of the filter (*migration and adhesion*). Which system reflects the *in vivo* situation is open to discussion, but it is important to realize their fundamental difference when discussing T lymphocyte migration *in vitro*.

It is also important to consider the relationship between "attraction" and "adhesion" as illustrated in Figure 1. It is seen that increased attraction may not necessarily lead to increased migration.

Cells must be handled with care (avoiding harsh centrifugations, resuspensions on vortex machines, cooling in refrigerators, etc.) and the handling must be absolutely standardized from experiment to experiment. Also, the time from blood drawing, isolation of cells and performance of the tests can be critical. Thus, if lymphocytes are left overnight before the chemotaxis assay is performed, they downregulate their IL-8 receptors [3], which can explain the observed differences alluded to above [1, 2].

The polyvinylpyrolidone filters must be of good quality without compounds that could be toxic to the cells and they should be coated with collagen to improve the assay's reproducibility. It is likely that further experiments on filter coating could improve both migration and adhesion studies of T lymphocytes as suggested in experiments in mice looking at amyloid A [4], basement membrane components [5] or β-2 integrins [6].

The size of the laser-induced holes in the filter is important. We have found 5 μm to be optimal, but it depends on the purity of cells, the amount of incubation time, etc. If one works with T cell lines of larger size such as blasts, the diameter may need to be different.

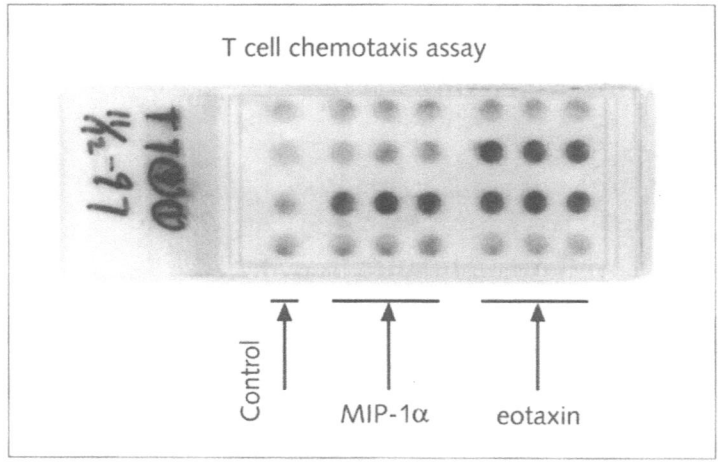

Figure 2
Picture of one chemotactic experiment performed with the Neuroprobe microwell tech-
nique. There are dose-response results from eotaxin and MIP-1α. It is easily seen how the
most stained wells were those showing the highest chemotactic index. Control wells are the
vertical wells on the left of each slide.

When performing the assay, one has to have a very steady hand when using the microwell system, because air bubles must be avoided when putting the medium with chemokine into the lower well of 25 μl volume. The filter must be carefully place to avoid air trapping. It is advisable to fixate the chamber body on a completely horisontal table in order to avoid unintended pushing. The upper part is then attached, secured, and then the upper chambers are fixed. Finally, the T lymphocyte population is gently put into the upper chambers of 25 μl – again avoiding air bubble formation.

On removal of the filter it should first be passed upside-down over a sharp rubber edge similar to a rubber policeman in order to remove cells on top of the filter. This must be done using forceps and gentle handling. Then the filter is slowly "washed" in saline, fixed in methanol and air-dried before staining with Coomassie blue. The filter is then dried and placed with the cells downwards on a glass slide. This allows a fixation where the slide and filter can be stored for months for documentation purposes (Fig. 2).

The reading of the number of cells can be done in a microscope, which is tedious, but will allow for single cell identification, or after staining with antibodies towards various phenotypes of the T lymphocytes. Today several systems can be used for computerized analysis of the cells. This also carries several considerations on how to avoid reading of debris, etc. Finally, the use of Coomassie blue combined with avoidance of debris and nonspecific binding of stain to the filters allows for a quick absorbance reading in an ELISA reader.

It is the experience of the authors that all steps above must be carefully considered and tested when using the T lymphocyte chemotaxis technique, and it may take up to 1 year to have tested all parameters. It is also necessary to perform checkerboard assays to differentiate between chemotaxis and chemokinesis [3].

If all these different parameters are not taken into consideration the results will not be suitable for publication.

T lymphocyte migration – experimental observations

It was first shown a decade ago that epidermal homogenates of suction blister roofs over a positive tuberculin skin reaction contained high-molecular weight (>8.000 dalton) compounds that were T lymphocyte chemotactic using the Boyden chamber technique [7]. It was also quickly realized the this chemotactic activity was directed towards CD4+ T lymphocytes [8].

Since then purified or recombinant peptides and not biological "homogenates" or supernatants have been the focus of attention with regard to T lymphocyte chemotaxis, one of the most studied being IL-8. At the moment (January, 1998) almost every issue of the *Journal of Immunology* (and many more journals) presents data on new T lymphocyte "chemokines" such as lymphotactin [9], IL-15 [10], IL-16 [11], MCP-1's to 3's [12], leukotactin-1 [13], PARC [14], fractalkine [15, 15a] and others [16].

Experimental observations using the Neuroprobe microwell technique

We have found the following observations which not only show some factual findings, but also indicate principal observations that could be significant in the interpretation of the *in vivo* situation. Again, most published literature at the moment – including our own – are *in vitro* observations. Few observations have been made *in vivo*.

Our observations are that many "chemokines" or other compounds such at LTB-4 induce "chemotaxis" of T lymphocytes. The chemotactic migration can at least be influenced *in vitro* by other cytokines – not necessarily chemokines, but also T cell growth factors – which will either promote (IFN-γ) or inhibit (IL-2 and IL-4) the effect of chemokines.

Figure 3 summarizes our findings: A majority of "pro-inflammatory" cytokines are T lymphocyte chemotactic (IL-1, IL-8 etc.). Some of these cytokines, such as

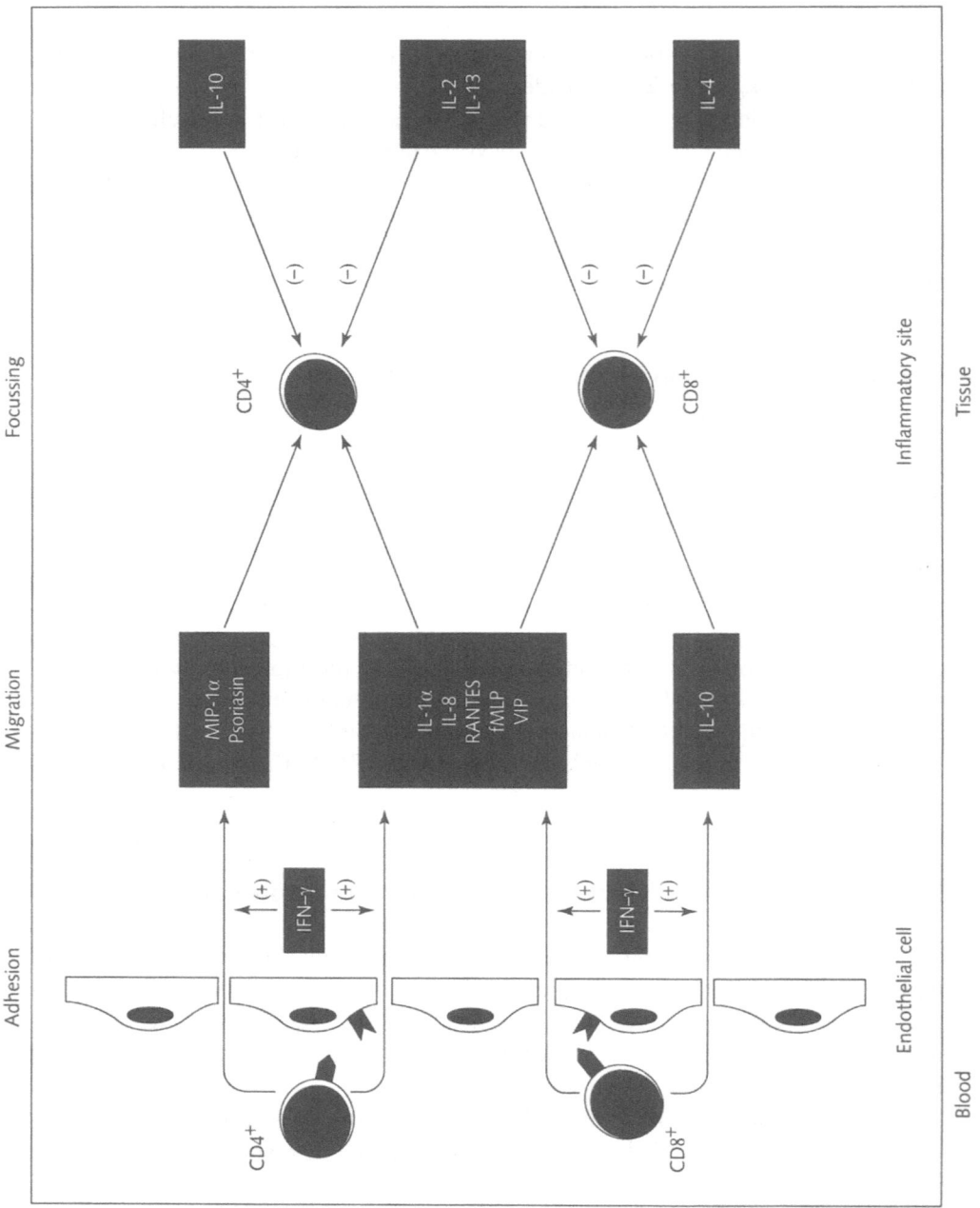

Figure 3
This diagram summarizes how various cytokines can influence T lymphocyte migration.

IL-8, are chemotactic to a broad range of leucocytes and may be important *in vivo* as indicators of tissue injury. Thus, oxygen-deprived cells will upregulate IL-8 (our own unpublished observations in HACAT keratinocytes; and [17]). Other chemokines may be more specific to various subsets of leucocytes. We observed how IL-10 is chemotactic to CD8[+] T lymphocytes [18], whereas a Ca^{2+}-binding peptide, psoriasin, is specifically chemotactic to CD4[+] T cells and neutrophil granulocytes, but not to CD8[+] T cells and monocytes [19]. We could not see that the T cell derived growth factors IL-2 and IL-4 are in themselves chemotactic, but they influence the ability of lymphocytes to respond to IL-8 and do so via regulation of the expression of IL-8 receptors. One of the important, specific T cell derived cytokines, IFN-γ, has a special capacity in augmenting the T cell response towards chemokines [3].

We have therefore put forward the concept of *migration and focussing*, i.e. when a T lymphocyte is "called" into an area of "tissue damage" it will enter. This migration can be augmented by IFN-γ i.e. if just a few T cells are activated in the area, then an increased migration takes place. When the migrating T cells meet T cell growth factors (Il-2 and Il-4), they "focus" in that area to continue their functions, i.e. they do not respond further to a proinflammatory cytokine such as IL-8 [3].

This concept would actually fit perfectly with the observations of Mechnikoff, who observed the forerunners (or the "anti-terrorist corps"), the granulocytes, but did not pay so much attention to the ensuing lymphocytic infiltration, which takes place in almost every "inflammatory" response. It is only when T cell derived factors become prominent that the T lymphocyte inflammation will be focused.

We have observed how the expression of chemokine receptors on B lymphocytes can be modulated by other pro-inflammatory cytokines or T cell growth factors [20]. We have also observed how healthy persons and HIV persons can differ in their capacity to upregulate IL-8 receptors. Specifically, we have observed – in B lymphocytes – that TNF-α could upregulate IL-8 receptors to a much more pronounced degree in B cells from HIV patients compared with normal persons [20].

Another observation illustrates the complexity in this field. We are at the moment studying T lymphocytes and their responsiveness towards various chemokines including eotaxin. Figure 4 shows how T cells are chemotactic to IL-8 and MIP-1α, but not to eotaxin (left figure). If, however, IL-2 and IL-4 is added to the lymphocytes during the assay, then the lymphocytes respond to eotaxin (right figure).

Thus, a very important issue, which is currently intensively studied, is the influence from *cytokines on chemokine receptor expression*. Future investigations will have to focus not only on this issue, but also on which *subtype of lymphocyte* responds to which cytokine, when considering chemokine receptor expression. At present, expression and regulation of chemokine receptors are at the center of interest because HIV uses these receptors for entering CD4[+] T lymphocytes [21]. The possiblity of pharmacological modulation of chemokine receptors is therefore an area of intense research. This review will not focus on this aspect of chemokines and

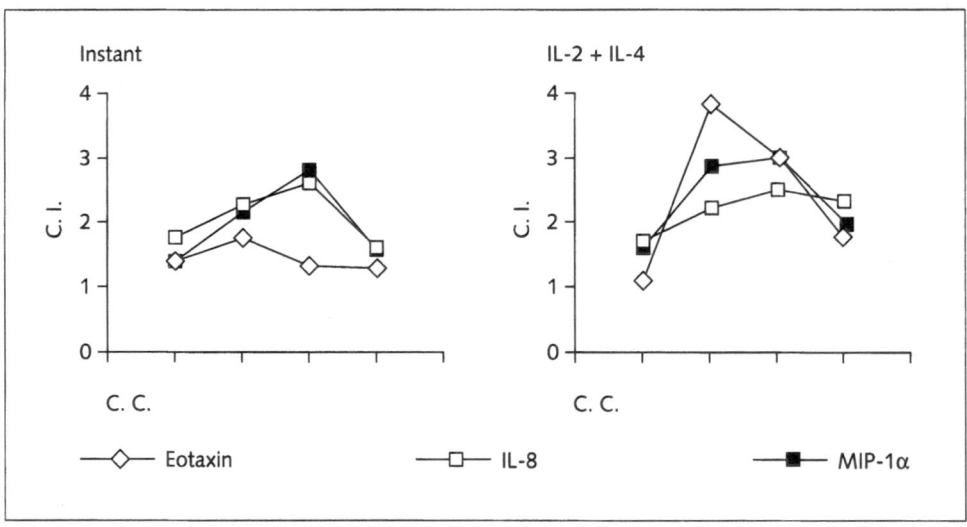

Figure 4
A representative experiment using peripheral blood T lymphocytes and their response to various cytokines. It is seen how incubation with IL-2 and IL-4 will induce a response towards eotaxin.

T lymphocytes, but readers are referred to excellent articles in this field [22–27]. The field of new knowledge about chemokine receptors including their cloning and expression is also expanding at a rapid pace [28–31].

In vitro **and** *in vivo* **observations**

A major issue when discussing chemokines and T lymphocyte migration is how much one can use the *in vitro* observations for understanding *in vivo* phenomena. Two examples are mentioned to elucidate this issue.

Psoriasin is a low-molecular weight Ca^{2+} binding molecule that is not listed under "chemokines", but was first isolated from "psoriatic epidermis". It was believed that psoriasin was only present in psoriatic skin, but it is also found in normal epidermis (J. Schröder, personal communication). We observed that psoriasin was chemotactic *in vitro* for CD4+ T lymphocytes and neutrophil granulocytes, but not for monocytes [19]. We then performed an *in vivo* experiment by inducing suction blisters in normal persons, injecting recombinant psoriasin into the blister (our own unpublished data). After 6 h, we took the cells in the blister for FACS analysis and also performed a biopsy of the underlying skin for histology. Figure 5 illustrates

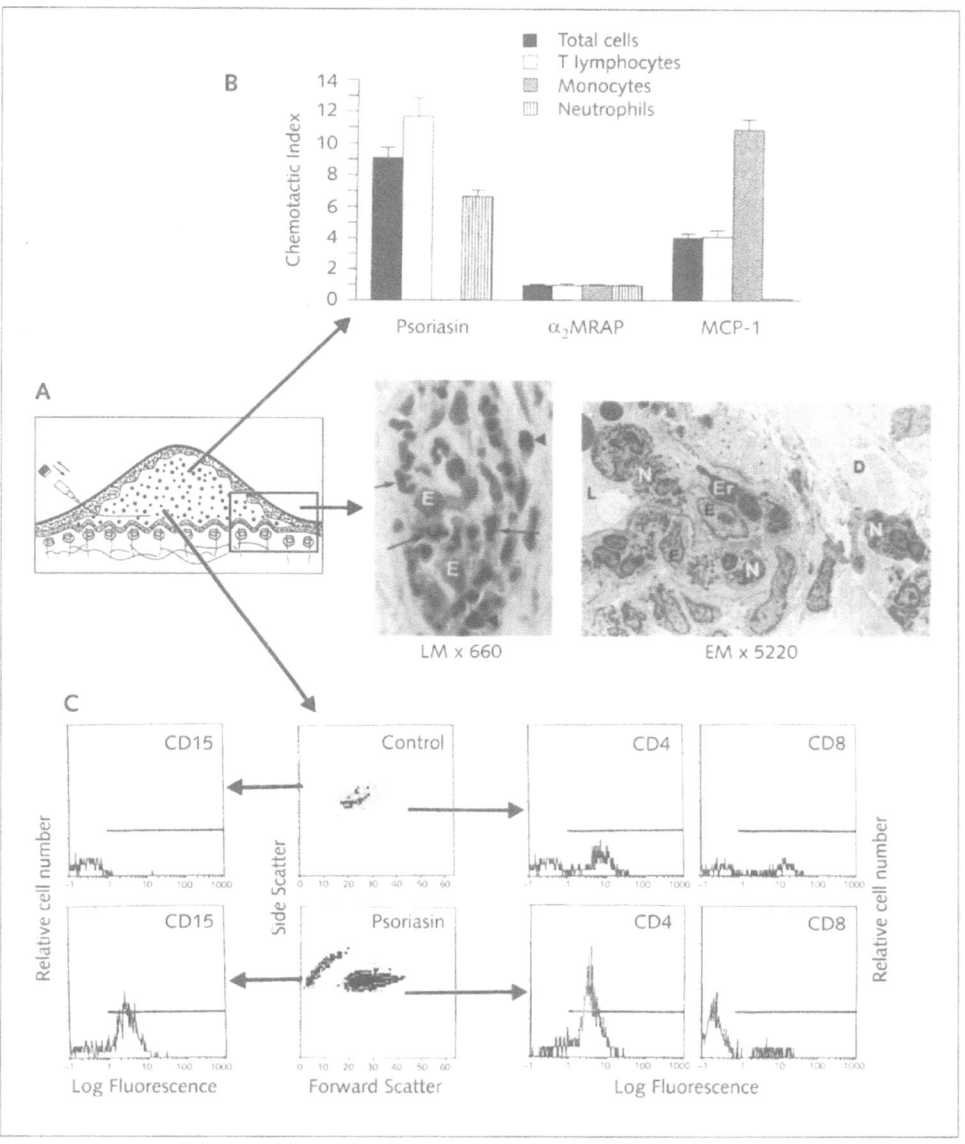

Figure 5
Results from studying the in vivo *effect of psoriasin in healthy volunteers. (A) the suction
blister; (B) the cells accumulated in the blister with psoriasin compared with alpha-2-MRAP,
a negative control, and MCP-1; (C) indicates the results of flow cytometry analyses of accu-
mulating cells in the blister with psoriasin and control blister. Additionally, biopsy observation after injection of psoriasin is also shown.*

our results. It is seen how both neutrophils and lymphocytes are present in the skin, and the FACS analysis confirmed that only neutrophil granulocytes and lymphocytes, but not monocytes were present. This *in vivo* observation thus illustrates how the *in vitro* observations are confirmed *in vivo* in an experimental setting.

Another example shows that this is not always so. Thus, we have observed how IL-10 is chemoattractant for CD8+ lymphocytes, but not for CD4+ T cells [18]. Dr. Sarvetnick and colleagues described in an intriguing series of experiments how they could couple the IFN-γ or IL-10 gene to the insulin promoter in a strain of mice [32]. When insulin was produced the mice either secreted IFN-γ or IL-10 and they observed that the IFN-γ-coupled mice developed type I diabetes, whereas the IL-10 mice developed "pancreatitis", i.e. lymphocyte mediated inflammation in the pancreas, but not diabetes (no cytotoxicity towards the β-cells). If our *in vitro* observations were "correct" biologically, then IFN-γ should lead to both CD4+ and CD8+ cellular infiltration, whereas IL-10 would mean a CD8+ T cell infiltration. However, this was not the case in these mice (S. Norvetnick, personal communication). Thus, there are many differences between *in vitro* and *in vivo* observations.

Sources of chemokines

There is no doubt that "chemokines" can arise from many cell types. Thus, IL-8 is likely to be secreted by any cell under "toxic" stress [17], and we have observed how mRNA for IL-8 can be upregulated in cells present in skin [33]. Recent observations confirm the plethora of possible influences from various tissue cells on accumulated cells from the immune system, if tissue damage occurs [34, 35].

How do T lymphocytes migrate?

Several studies have shown the role of "adhesion molecules" for T cell migration. There is no doubt that this issue is important for "T lymphocyte homing" (for reviews see [36–38]). There is an intimate relation between "chemokines" and "adhesion molecules" which is very relevant *in vivo* (see Fig. 3) [39]. This can be studied *in vitro* by coating the filters with different molecules relevant for T cell adhesion [40].

Recent studies have focused on proteolytic receptors such as the urokinase receptors being necessary for monocyte migration [41, 41a]. These receptors are also expressed on human T lymphocytes, but only on activated T lymphocytes [42]. We have not been able to detect them on migrating human freshly isolated T cells (unpublished). However, recent observations could demonstrate how the chemokine receptors CCR2 and CCR5 are at the leading front on migrating T lymphocytes [43]. This area needs further study.

Skin-homing T lymphocytes and chemokines

For years, immunologists have discussed the importance of "compartmentalization" of cells (for reviews see [36, 37]). It is most likely that T lymphocytes are equipped with different "keys" for various tissues – just like hotel guests have keys for their "compartments". Major focus has been put on cutaneous lymphocyte antigen, which may be an important "adhesion molecule" for skin-homing T cells [44–48]. It will be of interest to see if chemokines regulate the epitope expression of CLA.

We are in the process of describing how skin-homing T lymphocytes can show cytokine-driven, but antigen-independent, *in vitro* growth when put into culture with high amounts of the cytokines IL-2 and IL-4 (Bang et al., in preparation). These T cell cultures are polyclonal in their growth, and they do show ability to respond to various chemokines – including eotaxin (see Fig. 4). The growth capacity of skin-homing T lymphocytes is different from blood T lymphocytes from the same patient, thus directly demonstrating a significant functional difference.

In vivo models for the importance of chemokines and cytokines

New and probably biologically relevant observations are now achieved through injection of antibodies towards proinflammatory cytokines. Thus, we have shown how IL-8 is a significant contributor in the development of the tuberculin skin reaction [49]. Knock-out mice or transgenic mice are also interesting models. MIP-1α -/- mice cannot establish an appropriate inflammation towards Coxsackievirus-induced myocarditis [50], and mice lacking the IL-8 receptors develop neutrophila [51] and have problems with the regulation of myeloid progenitor cells *in vivo* [52,53]. Also, if eotaxin cannot be normally expressed this will reduce tissue eosinophilia following antigen provocation [54]. Another recent study showed how important chemokine receptors may be in normal homeostasis [55]. Finally, transgenic mice overexpressing the T cell growth factor, IL-7, in their keratinocytes will develop "lymphoproliferative skin disease" [56].

Conclusion and perspectives

No doubt researchers are looking at many *in vitro* experiments which demonstrate the redundancy in biological systems. It is likely that most of what we see *in vitro* is not relevant *in vivo*. However, the *in vitro* models for T lymphocyte migration are necessary paths to get information about new peptides and their possible biological roles. This allows for the design of biological models of interest.

A fundamental question is whether the T lymphocytes creating tissue inflammation are just blood T lymphocytes called in by chemokines, or they do have specific properties that have not been studied so far? The authors believe that, apart from their migratory capacities tissue-homing, inflammatory T lymphocytes have many functions that are so far unknown. It is possible that the reason some persons can create inflammation as seen in chronic inflammatory diseases of various organs (skin, lung, joints, intestine) may relate to the developement of tissue-specific T lymphocytes that have not been described so far [57, 58]. It will be exciting to discover such populations of inflammatory cells and learn their differences from circulating T lymphocytes.

Acknowledgements
The authors wish to express their sincere thanks to the following foundations and institutions for support of the research work: Alfred Benzon Fond, Aarhus University Foundation, Aage Bangs Fond, the Danish Medical Research Council, Institute of Clinical and Experimental Research, Novo-Nordisk Foundation, and Velux Fonden.

References

1   Larsen CG, Anderson AO, Appella E, Oppenheim JJ, Matsushima K (1989) Neutrophil activating factor (NAP-1) is also chemotactic for T lymphocytes. *Science* 243: 1464–1468

2   Taub DD, Conlon K, Lloyd AR, Oppenheim JJ, Kelvin DJ (1993) Preferential migration of activated CD8+ and CD4+ T cells in response to MIP-1-α and MIP-1-β. *Science* 260: 355–357

3   Jinquan T, Deleuran B, Gesser B, Maare H, Deleuran M, Larsen CG, Thestrup-Pedersen K (1995) Regulation of Human T lymphocyte chemotaxis *in vitro* by T cell-derived cytokines IL-2, IFN-gamma, IL-4, IL-10, and IL-13. *J Immunol* 154; 3742–3752.

4   Xu L, Badolato R, Murphy WJ, Longo DL, Anver M, Hale S, Oppenheim JJ, Wang JM (1995) A novel biologic function of serum amyloid A. Induction of T lymphocyte migration and adhesion. *J Immunol* 155: 1184–1190

5   Li Y-Y, Cheung HT (1992) Basement membrane and its components on lymphocyte adhesion, migration, and proliferation. *J Immunol* 149: 3174–3184

6   Somersalo K, Tarkkanen J, Patarroyo M, Saksela E (1992) Involvement of β-2-integrins in the migration of human natural killer cells. *J Immunol* 149: 590–598

7   Ternowitz T, Thestrup-Pedersen K (1986) Epidermis and lymphocyte interactions during a tuberculin skin reaction. II. Homogenized epidermal tissue supernatant has increased chemotactic activity for lymphocytes. *J Invest Dermatol* 87: 613–617

8   Zachariae C, Ternowitz T, Larsen CG, Nielsen V, Thestrup-Pedersen K (1988) Epidermal lymphocyte chemotactic factor specifically attracts OKT4 positive lymphocytes. *Arch Dermatol Res* 280: 354–357

9   Kelner GS, Kennedy J, Bacon KB, Kleyensteuber S, Largaespade DA, Jenkins NA, Copeland NG, Banan JF, Moore KW, Schall TJ, Zlotnik A (1994) Lymphotactin: A cytokine that represents a new class of chemokine. *Science* 266: 1395–1399

10 Wilkinson PC, Liew FY (1995) Chemoattraction of human blood T lymphocytes by interleukin-15. *J exp Med* 181: 1255–1259

11 Laberge S, Cruikshank WW, Beer DJ, Center DM (1996) Secretion of IL-16 (lymphocyte chemoattractant factor) from serotonin-stimulated CD8$^+$ T cells *in vitro. J Immunol* 156: 310–315

12 Taub DD, Proost P, Murphy WJ, Anver M, Longo DL, Damme JV, Oppenheim JJ (1995) Monocyte chemotactic protein-1 (MCP-1), -2, and -3 are chemotactic for human T lymphocytes. *J Clin Invest* 95: 1370–1376

13 Youn B-S, Zhang SM, Lee EK, Park DH, Broxmeyer HE, Murphy PM, Locati M, Pease JE, Kim KK, Antol K, Kwon BS (1997) Molecular cloning of leukotactin-1: A novel human β-chemokine, a chemoattractant for neutrophils, monocytes, and lymphocytes, and a potent agonist at CC chemokine receptors 1 and 3. *J Immunol* 159: 5201–5205

14 Hieshima K, Imai T, Baba M, Shoudai K, Ishizuka K, Nakagawa T, Tsuruta J, Takeya M, Sakaki Y, Takatsuki K, Miura R, Opdenakker G, Damme JV, Yoshie O, Nomiyama H (1997) A novel human CC chemokine PARC that is most homologous to macrophage-inflammatory protein-1α/LD78α and chemotactic for T lymphocytes, but not for monocytes. *J Immunol* 159: 1140–1149

15 Schall T (1997) Fractalkine – strange attractor in the chemokine landscape. *Immunol Today* 19: 147

15a Bazan JF, Bacon KB, Hardiman G, Wang W, Soo K, Rossi D, Greaves DR, Zlotnik A, Schall TJ (1997) A new class of membrane-bound chemokine with a CX3C motif. *Nature* 385: 640–644.

16 Hedrick JA, Zlotnick A (1997) Identification and characterization of a novel β-chemokine containing six conserved cysteines. *J Immunol* 159: 1589–1593

17 Desbaillets I, Diserens A-C, Tribolet N, Hamou M-F, van Meir EG (1997) Upregulation of interleukin 8 by oxygen-deprived cells in glioblastoma suggests a role in leukocyte activation, chemotaxis, and angiogenesis. *J exp Med* 186: 1201–1212

18 Jinquan T, Larsen CG, Gesser B, Matsushima K, Thestrup-Pedersen K (1993) Human interleukin 10 is a chemoattractant for CD8$^+$ T lymphocytes and an inhibitor of CD4$^+$ T lymphocyte migration. *J Immunol* 151: 4545–4551

19 Jinquan T, Vorum H, Larsen CG, Gesser B, Rasmussen HH, Madsen PB, Honoré B, Etzerodt M, Nielsen V, Celis JE, Thestrup-Pedersen K (1996) Psoriasin: A novel chemotactic protein. *J Invest Dermatol* 107: 5–10

20 Jinquan T, Møller B, Storgaard M, Mukaida N, Bonde J, Grunnet N, Black FT, Larsen CG, Matsushima K, Thestrup-Pedersen K (1997) Chemotaxis and IL-8 receptor expression in B cells from normal and HIV-infected subjects. *J Immunol* 158: 475–484

21 Wu L, LaRosa G, Kassam N, Gordon CJ, Heath H, Ruffing N, Chen H, Humblias J, Samson M, Parmentier M, Moore JP, Mackay CR (1997) Interaction of chemokine

receptor CCR5 with its ligands: Multiple domains for HIV-1 gp120 binding and a single domain for chemokine binding. *J exp Med* 186: 1373–1381

22   Oravecz T, Pall M, Norcross MA (1996) β-chemokine inhibition of monocytotropic HIV-1 infection. Interference with a postbinding fusion step. *J Immunol* 157: 1329–1332

23   Verani A, Scarlatti G, Comar M, Tresoldi E, Polo S, Giacca M, Lusso P, Siccardi AG, Vercelli D (1997) CC chemokines released by lipopolysaccharide (LPS)-stimulated human macrophages suppress HIV-1 infection in both macrophages and T cells. *J exp Med* 185: 805–816

24   Amara A, Gall SL, Schwartz O, Salamero J, Montes M, Loetscher P, Baggiolini M, Virelizier J-L, Arenzana-Sesdedos F (1997) HIV coreceptor downregulation as antiviral principle: SDF-1α-dependent internalization of the chemokine receptor CXCR4 contributes to inhibition of HIV replication. *J exp Med* 186: 139–146

25   Doranz BJ, Grovit-Ferbas K, Sharron MP, Mao S-H, Goetz MB, Daar ES, Doms RW, O'Brien WA (1997) A small-molecule inhibitor directed against the chemokine receptor CXCR4 prevents its use as an HIV-1 coreceptor. *J exp Med* 186: 1395–1400

26   Murakami T, Nakajima T, Koyanagi Y, Tachibana K, Fujii N, Tamamura H, Yoshida N, Waki M, Matsumoto A, Yoshie O, Hishimoto T, Yamamoto N, Nagasawa T (1997) A small molecule CXCR4 inhibitor that blocks T cell line-tropic HIV-1 infection. *J exp Med* 186: 1389–1393

27   Schols D, Struyf S, van Damme J, Esté JA, Henson G, de Clercq E (1997) Inhibition of T-tropic HIV strains by selective antagonization of the chemokine receptor CXCR4. *J exp Med* 186: 1383–1388

28   Post TW, Bozic CR, Rothenberg ME, Luster AD, Gerard N, Gerard C (1995) Molecular characterization of two murine eosinophil β-chemokine receptors. *J Immunol* 155: 5299–5305

29   Greaves DR, Wang W, Dairaghi DJ, Dieu MC, de Saint-Vis B, Franz-Bacon K, Rossi D, Caux C, McClanahan T, Gordon S, Zlotnik A, Schall TJ (1997) CCR6, a CC chemokine receptor that interacts with macrophage inflammatory protein 3α and is highly expressed in human dendritic cells. *J exp Med* 186: 837–844

30   Power CA, Church DJ, Meyer A, Alouani S, Proudfoot AEI, Clark-Lewis I, Sozzani S, Mantovani A, Wells TNC (1997) Cloning and characterization of a specific receptor for the novel CC chemokine MIP-3α from lung dendritic cells. *J exp Med* 186: 825–835

31   Tiffany HL, Lautens LL, Gao J-L, Pease J, Locati M, Combadiere C, Modi W, Bonner TI, Murphy PM (1997) Identification of CCR8: A human monocyte and thymus receptor for the CC chemokine I-309. *J exp Med* 186: 165–170

32   Wogensen L, Huang X, Sarvetnick N (1993) Leukocyte extravasation into the pancreatic tissue in transgenic mice expressing interleukin-10 in the islets of Langerhans. *J exp Med* 178: 175–185

33   Kristensen M, Paludan K, Larsen CG, Zachariae C, Deleuran B, Jensen PKA, Jørgensen P, Thestrup-Pedersen K (1991) Quantitative determination of IL-1alfa-induced IL-8 mRNA levels in cultured human keratinocytes, dermal fibroblasts, endothelial cells, and monocytes. *J Invest Dermatol* 97: 506–510

34   Rumsaeng V, Cruikshank WW, Foster B, Prussin C, Kirshenbaum AS, Davis TA, Korn-feld H, Center DM, Metcalfe DD (1997) Human mast cells produce the CD4$^+$ T lymphocyte chemoattractant factor, IL-16. *J Immunol* 159: 2904–2910

35   Stoll S, Müller G, Kurimoto M, Saloga J, Tanimoto T, Yamauchi H, Okamura H, Knop J, Enk AH. Production of IL-18 (IFN-γ-inducing factor) messenger RNA and functional protein by murine keratinocytes. *J Immunol* 1997 159: 298–302

36   Picker LJ 1992) Mechanisms of lymphocyte homing. *Curr Opin Immunol* 4: 277–286

37   Issekutz TB (1992) Lymphocyte homing to sites of inflammation. *Curr Opin Immunol* 4: 287–293

38   Downey GP (1994) Mechanisms of leukocyte motility and chemotaxis. *Curr Opin Immunol* 6: 113–124

39   Zimmerman GA, McIntyre TM, Prescott SM (1996) Adhesion and signaling in vascular cell-cell interactions. *J Clin Invest* 98: 1699–1702

40   Hauzenberger D, Klominek J, Sundqvist K-G (1994) Functional specialization of fibronectin-binding β-1-integrins in T lymphocyte migration. *J Immunol* 153: 960–971

41   Gyetko MR, Todd III RF, Wilkinson CC, Sitrin RG (1994) The urokinase receptor is required for human monocyte chemotaxis *in vitro*. *J Clin Invest* 93: 1380–1387

41a Blasi F (1997) uPA, uPAR, PAI-I: key intersection of proteolytic, adhesive and chemotactic highways? *Immunol Today* 18: 415–417

42   Nykjaer A, Møller B, Todd RF III, Christensen T, Andreasen PA, Gliemann J, Petersen CM (1994) Urokinase receptor. An activation antigen in human T lymphocytes. *J Immunol* 152: 505–516

43   Nieto M, Frade JMR, Sancho D, Mellado M, Martinez-A C, Sánches-Madrid F (1997) Polarization of chemokine receptors to the leading edge during lymphocyte chemotaxis. *J exp Med* 186: 153–158

44   Bos JD, de Boer OJ, Tibosch E, Das PK, Pals ST (1993) Skin-homing T lymphocytes: detection of cutaneous lymphocyte associated antigen (CLA) by HECA-452 in normal human skin. *Arch Dermatol Res* 285: 179–183

45   Leung DYM, Gately M, Trumble A, Ferguson-Darnell B, Schlievert PM, Picker LJ (1995) Bacterial superantigens induce T cell expression of the skin-selective homing receptor, the cutaneous lymphocyte-associated antigen, via stimulation of interleukin 12 production. *J exp Med* 181: 747–753

46   Babi LFS, Moser R, Soler MTP, Picker LJ, Blaser K, Hauser C (1995) Migration of skin-homing T cells across cytokine-activated human endothelial cell layers involves interaction of the cutaneous lymphocyte-associated antigen (CLA), the very late antigen-4 (VLA-4), and the lymphocyte function-associated antigen-1 (LFA-1). *J Immunol* 154: 1543–1550

47   Kunstfeld R, Lechleitner S, Gröger M, Wolff K, Petzelbauer P (1997) HECA-452 T cells migrate through superficial vascular plexus but not through deep vascular plexus endothelium. *J Invest Dermatol* 108: 343–348

48   Fuhlbrigge RC, Kieffer JD, Armerding D, Kupper TS (1997) Cutaneous lymphocyte

antigen is a specialized form of PSGL-1 expressed on skin-homing T cells. *Nature* 389: 978–981

49 Larsen CG, Thomsen MK, Gesser B, Thomsen PD, Deleuran BW, Nowak J, Skødt V, Thomsen KH, Deleuran M, Thestrup-Pedersen K, Harada A, Matsushima K, Menné T (1995) The delayed-type hypersensitivity reaction is dependent on IL-8. Inhibition of a tuberculin skin reaction by an anti-IL-8 monoclonal antibody. *J Immunol* 155: 2151–2157

50 Cook DN, Beck MA, Coffman TM, Kirby SL, Sheridan JF, Pragnell IB, Smithies O (1995) Requirement of MIP-1α for an inflammatory response to viral infection. *Science* 269: 1583–1585

51 Schuster DE, Kehrli ME, Ackermann MR (1995) Neutrophilia in mice that lack the murine IL-8 receptor homolog. *Science* 269: 1590–1591

52 Broxmeyer HE, Cooper S, Cacalano G, Hague NL, Bailish E, Moore MW (1996) Involvement of interleukin (IL) 8 receptor in negative regulation of myeloid progenitor cells *in vivo*: Evidence from mice lacking the murine IL-8 receptor homologue. *J exp Med* 184: 1825–1832

53 Nagasawa T, Hirota S, Tachibana K, Takakura N, Nishikawa S-I, Kitamura Y, Yoshida N, Kikutani H, Kishimoto T (1996) Defects of B-cell lymphopoiesis and bone-marrow myelopoiesis in mice lacking the CXC chemokine PBSF/SDF-1. *Nature* 382: 635–638

54 Rothenberg ME, MacLean JA, Pearlman E, Luster AD, Leder P (1997) Targeted disruption of the chemokine eotaxin partially reduces antigen-induced tissue eosinophilia. *J exp Med* 185: 785–790

55 Kuziel WA, Morgan SJ, Dawson TC, Friffin S, Smithies O, Ley K, Maeda N (1997) Severe reduction in leukocyte adhesion and monocyte extravasation in mice deficient in CC chemokine receptor 2. *Proc Natl Acad Sci USA* 94: 12053–12058

56 Williams IF, Rawson EA, Manning L, Karaoli T, Rich BE, Kupper TS (1997) IL-7 overexpression in transgenic mouse keratinocytes causes a lymphoproliferative skin disease dominated by intermedidate TCR cells. Evidence for a hierarchy in IL-7 responsiveness among cutaneous T cells. *J Immunol* 159: 3044-3056

57 Thestrup-Pedersen K, Ellingsen AR, Olesen AB, Kaltoft K (1997) Atopic dermatitis may be a genetically determined dysmaturation of ectodermal tissue resulting in disturbed T lymphocyte maturation. A hypothesis. *Acta Dermato-venereol* (Stockh) 77: 20–21

58. Thestrup-Pedersen K (1997) Which factors are of importance in the pathophysiology of atopic dermatitis. *Eur J Dermatol* 7: 549–553

Chemokines and mast cells

Sabine Krüger-Krasagakes[1], Andreas Grützkau[1], Undine Lippert[2] and Beate M. Henz[1]

[1]Department of Dermatology, Charité-Virchow Clinic, Humboldt University, Augustenburger Platz 1, D-13344 Berlin, Germany
[2]Department of Dermatology, University Hospital, von-Siebold-Strasse 3, D-37075 Göttingen, Germany

Basic mast cell properties

Mast cells derive from bone marrow stem cells, are ubiquitously distributed resident tissue cells, and are particularly frequent in the lamina propria of epithelial organs, including the skin. The cells are characterized and distinguishable from other cells by their electrondense cytoplasmatic granules, their contents of mediators like histamine, heparin and tryptase, and by their surface receptors for SCF (c-kit) and IgE (the high affinity IgE receptor, FcεRI). Basophils which belong to the granulocytic series of the bone marrow and reside primarily in peripheral blood, are often grouped with mast cells since they share many properties with these cells except for their morphology and their lack of tryptase and c-kit. Mast cells also have a number of properties in common with other tissue resident and infiltrating inflammatory cells like the receptors c-kit on melanocytes, FcεRI on Langerhans cells, and C3bR, C5aR and FcγRIII on monocytes and granulocytes. Furthermore, like most inflammatory cells, they are able to produce a broad range of mediators including leukotrienes, platelet activating factor (PAF) and cytokines. While mast cells have traditionally been viewed as primary effector cells of immediate type allergic reactions, their potential role in diverse other immunological and inflammatory processes has become more and more apparent in recent years (for review, see [1]).

Thus, it is well established that mast cell-dependent inflammation, as classically represented by urticaria in the skin, is not only characterized by vasodilatation and edema, but also by inflammatory infiltrates. As recently shown by us in a large series of urticaria patients comparing normal and involved skin, this infiltrate consists of neutrophils, eosinophils and their products as well as activated macrophages and lymphocytes, with an associated increase of mast cells [2, 3]. The mast cell-derived mediators possibly inducing the influx of these cells have long been thought to represent primarily the low molecular weight lipid mediators leukotriene (LT) B_4 and PAF [4]. In fact, elevated levels of LTB_4 have been demonstrated in lesional skin of urticaria [5]. Via activation by mast cell constituents, complement components like C3a and C5a might also contribute to tissue edema and the inflammatory infiltrate [4].

Evidence that additional types of mediators might be involved in mast cell-dependent inflammation came from the demonstration of high molecular weight neutrophil chemotactic factors, released from mast cells and basophils on antigen-dependent challenge *in vitro* [6, 7] and in the venous effluent blood close to sites of challenge in patients with cold urticaria [8]. With the demonstration of cytokine production by murine mast cells [9] and the detection of chemotactic cytokines, now grouped into the chemokine families of molecules, we reasoned that mast cells might produce chemokines and indeed succeeded in demonstrating this for the first time with IL-8 [10]. Since then, a number of additional findings in our laboratory and data published recently in the literature have expanded the body of knowledge on the relationship of mast cells and chemokines. The present review will summarize the data available so far regarding both chemokine production and secretion by mast cells, and conversely, the effect of these molecules on mast cells. Finally, the potential significance of these findings in cutaneous disease will be discussed.

Mast cell-derived chemokines

CXC chemokines

From among all mast cell-derived chemokines, IL-8 has been most extensively studied (Tab. 1). Its expression was first demonstrated by us in stimulated murine PB3c and RBL cell lines [11] and subsequently in human leukemic HMC-1 cells [10]. Since it is extremely difficult to isolate sufficient quantities of purified tissue mast cells, the HMC-1 cells proved to be a valuable alternative for study, also since they closely resemble normal human mast cells, including even the variable expression of the FcεRI [12, 13].

In the absence of any stimulus, IL-8 mRNA was not detected at all [10] or at very low levels [14]. Stimulation of the cells with the ionophore A23187 or phorbol myristate acetate (PMA) caused a dose-dependent upregulation of IL-8 message and the combined stimulation was even more effective. Other stimuli like IL-1α or β, LPS or a sequence of passive sensitisation with IgE and anti-IgE were ineffective in HMC-1 cells. Studies of the kinetics of IL-8 mRNA expression on A23187/PMA stimulation showed that upregulation was evident already by 1 h, reaching maximal levels by 6–8 h, with still detectable levels at 48 h [10, 14]. Comparative studies with a number of cytokines and growth factors yielded very different kinetics for the different molecules and underlined the particularly extended kinetics of IL-8 mRNA, suggesting that stabilizing processes or inhibition of mRNA degrading enzymes might be operative [14]. Cycloheximide had no effect on IL-8 mRNA transcription,

Table 1 - Expression of mRNA and production of chemokines by murine and human mast cells

	Murine mc*	Tissue mc	HMC-1	mRNA	
				constitutive	stimulated
CXC chemokines					
IL-8	+	+	+	−**	+
MARC	+	−	−	−	+
CC chemokines					
I-309			+	+	+
MCP-1			+	+	+
MCP-5	−		+	−	+
MIP-1α			+	−	+
MIP-1β			+	−	+
RANTES			+	−	+
C-chemokines					
Ltn	+		+	−	+

* mc = mast cells

** In an earlier study [10] and in one from another group [18], preformed IL-8 mRNA was not found, but a later passage of the leukemic cells exhibited IL-8 mRNA already prior to stimulation [14].

in contrast to IL-6 mRNA, whereas treatment of the cells with actinomycin D was stabilizing [14], indicating that IL-8 is regulated as a primary response gene and that additional posttranscriptional regulatory mechanisms are operative. In studies of HMC-1 cells by another group, IL-4 was shown to enhance ionomycin-stimulated IL-8 mRNA by about fourfold [15].

In culture supernatants of stimulated HMC-1 cells, only a single 8 kD molecule was detected on immunoblot with an anti-IL-8 antibody. These findings were identical to those observed with the monocytic cell line THP1 which was studied for comparison [10]. The kinetics of secretion, as studied by ELISA, showed detectable levels of IL-8 already by 2 h (0.3–1.3 ng/ml/10^6 cells), with increasing levels up to the last time point studied (72 h) (Fig. 1). The highest levels reached (53.2 ng/ml/10^6 cells) exceeded by at least one order of magnitude the highest levels of other cytokines measured in the same experimental setting [10, 14]. Secretion of IL-8 was inhibitable by up to 80% by corticosteroids and by up to 50% with the active

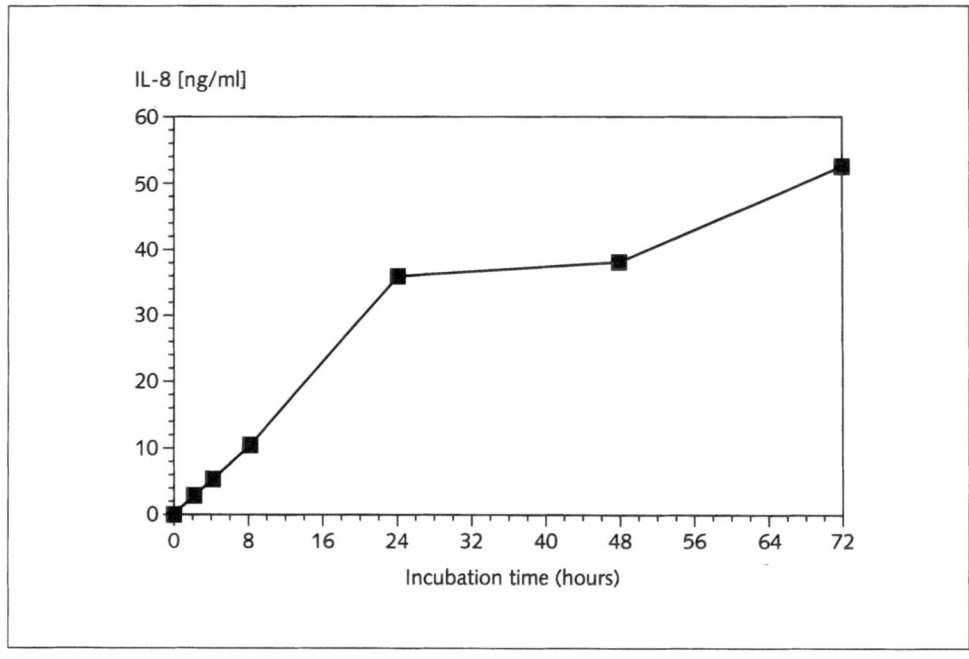

Figure 1
Time-dependent release of IL-8 from stimulated HMC-1 cells. For experimental details, see text and [14].

metabolite of a new generation H1-antagonist, descarboethoxy-loratadine, although the latter was only active after a 1-h preincubation with HMC-1 cells, whereas dexamethasone was inhibitory also when added to the cells together with the stimulus [16].

Functional studies provided evidence that IL-8 in HMC-1 cell culture supernatants was able to induce human neutrophil chemotaxis, with activities almost twice those of rhIL-8 at 50 ng/ml [10]. Inhibition of this activity with an anti-IL-8 antibody were however not complete (our own unpublished data), suggesting that additional neutrophil chemotactic molecules were secreted by HMC-1 cells.

IL-8 could also be demonstrated intracellularly in up to 50% of stimulated HMC-1 cells by immunocytochemistry, and by flow cytometry of permeabilized cells [17]. On immunoelectron microscopy, IL-8 was localized to the cytoplasmatic granules of stimulated HMC-1 cells (Fig. 2). Also after *in vitro* incubation of normal human skin with IgE and anti-IgE, IL-8 was detected on intracellular membranous structures and granules of stimulated, but not on mast cells of unstimulated skin, as determined by immunoelectron microscopy [10].

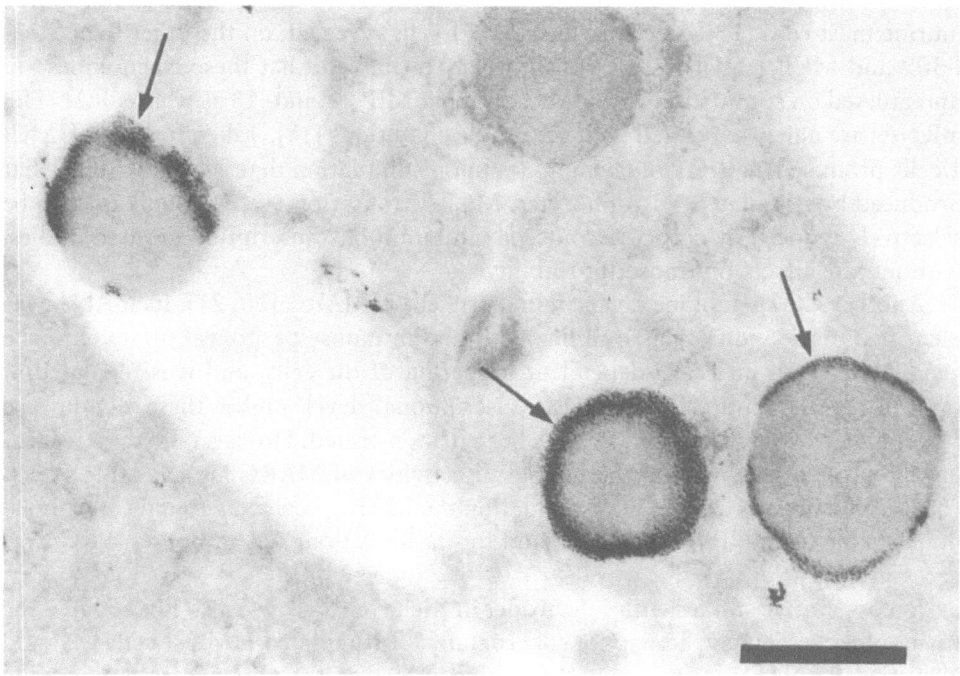

Figure 2
Pre-embedding immunoelectron microscopy of HMC-1 cells stimulated for 8 h with
0.25 μM calcium ionophore A23187 and 25 ng/ml PMA. Immunolabeling for IL-8 was visu-
alized by a silver enhanced secondary 1-nm gold conjugated anti-mouse IgG [17]. IL-8-spe-
cific immunostaining was most frequently observed at the periphery of cytoplasmic granules
(arrows). Bar: 0.5 μm.

Moreover, double-staining of biopsy specimens from patients with various types of cutaneous diseases showed that between 5–19% of mast cells reacted for IL-8, with particularly increased staining in the deep dermis of delayed pressure urticaria (our own unpublished data).

CC chemokines

The potential production of this group of chemokines by mast cells has so far been studied only at the mRNA level except for I-309 and MCP-1, which have been described as proteins [18]. The mediators are not invariably expressed on mast cells since the recently described MCP-5 was not detected in two types of activated murine mast cells [19]. Screening of HMC-1 cells revealed, on the other hand, that I-309 and MCP-1 mRNAs are constitutively expressed, that these chemokines are upregulated on stimulation with PMA, and that MIP-1α and -1β as well as RANTES mRNAs are newly expressed under the same conditions [18]. Taken together, HMC-1 cells produced an array of chemokines upon stimulation that is broader than that produced by stimulated T lymphocytes. MCP-1 transcripts were the only ones to be selectively reduced by corticosteroids via inhibition of transcription in these studies, without any effects on transcript stability.

Another CC chemokine detected in mast cells is MARC [20, 21]. Its mRNA was identified in the mouse mast cell line CPII and in mouse peritoneal mast cells. The gene is activated on FcεRI-dependent triggering of the cells, and it is regulated at both the transcriptional and posttranscriptional level under these conditions. Homologies with MCP-1 and -2 have been demonstrated. However, no data regarding the protein product and the biological activities of MARC are available as yet. An AP3-like transcription factor regulating the MARC gene was found to be indistinguishable from NF-AT in T cells, and for its activation, p21[ras], but not PKC, was necessary [22].

In cooperative studies with J. Schröder in Kiel, Germany, we also investigated the eosinophil chemotactic activity of supernatants of stimulated HMC-1 cells [23] and identified RANTES as the main chemokine. Whether the C-C chemokine eotaxin and other eosinophil chemotactic chemokines like MIP-1α contribute to this activity will have to be further clarified.

The C-chemokine lymphotactin (Ltn)

Very recently, the expression of a novel chemokine with supposedly only lymphocyte chemotatic properties, Ltn, was demonstrated in HMC-1 cells and in cultured murine mast cells after FcεRI-dependent or ionomycin stimulation [24]. Its transcription was inhibited by cyclosporin A and dexamethasone, and enhanced by TGF-β and IL-4. The presence of Ltn protein was demonstrated intracellularly and in culture supernatants. No further data are available regarding the secretion, structure or function of mast cell-derived Ltn.

Mast cell response to chemokines

Chemokine receptors

Since chemokines are known to potentially induce diverse functions in different cell types, we reasoned that these molecules might also have such effects on mast cells.

Since the first step in the mediation of such activities generally occurs via surface receptors, we first turned to the study of IL-8 receptors.

Apart from a report on IL-8 binding to human perivascular skin mast cells [25], no other data on possible chemokine receptors on mast cells are available so far. In various other cells, two types of IL-8 receptors have however so far been identified and characterized, a CXCR1 receptor, formerly called type A receptor, which binds IL-8 with high affinity, and its structural analogues MGSA and NAP-2 with low affinity, and a CXCR2 (type B) receptor which binds all three molecules with high affinity [26].

In a series of experiments, we set out to study these receptors on HMC-1 and on normal human skin mast cells. Both receptors were readily detectable on unstimulated HMC-1 cells at the mRNA level [27]. With the use of specific antibodies, about 70% of HMC-1 cells expressed the CXCR1 and 15% the CXCR2 on their cell membrane by flow cytometry. Using immunoelectron microscopical methods and the same antibodies to study normal human skin mast cells, CXCR1 was detctable mainly on the cell membrane and narrow surface folds (Fig. 3A) whereas CXCR2 was detected solely on specific cytoplasmatic mast cell granules and in the nucleus (Fig. 3B) [28]. Scatchard plot analyses revealed both high and low affinity binding sites for IL-8 and for MGSA on HMC-1 cells, but there were about tenfold more binding sites for IL-8 than for MGSA [28]. Nevertheless, studies on intracellular calcium mobilization showed both IL-8 and MGSA to be about equally active and NAP-2 to be a weaker stimulus [27]. Taken together, these data suggest that IL-8 receptor expression is heterogeneous and that additional IL-8 binding sites are possibly present on mast cells.

Chemokines and mast cell chemotaxis

As would be expected from the demonstration of the IL-8 receptors on mast cells and the potency of the chemotactic response induced by IL-8 in other cells, rhIL-8, MGSA and NAP-2 caused a dose-dependent *in vitro* chemotactic (directed) and chemokinetic (undirected) migration of both HMC-1 and human skin mast cells, with an optimal response at about 10^{-8} M concentrations [27, 28]. This activity was accompanied by a rapid increase of intracellular free calcium and an induction of actin polymerization, a basic prerequisite for cell migration [27].

Apart from these studies, *in vitro* chemotactic responsiveness of human mast cells has been observed only with RANTES, using cultured human cord blood-derived mast cells. MCP-1, MIP-1α and MIP-1β were inactive in these same studies [29]. Unstimulated murine bone marrow-derived mast cells responded on the other hand to MCP-1 and RANTES [30], and prestimulation with IgE, MCP-1, MIP-1α and PF4 induced a chemotactic reponse in the same cells [30].

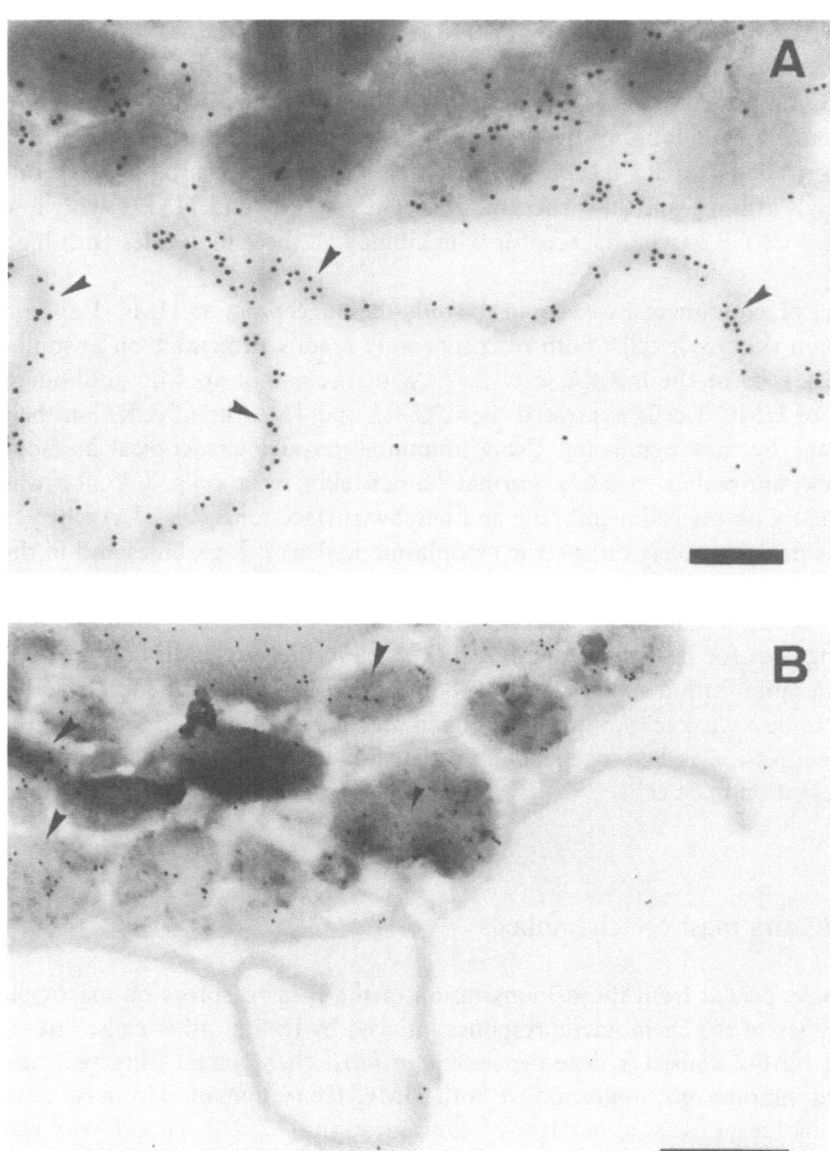

Figure 3
Immunoelectron microscopic localization of IL-8 receptors on ultra-thin sections of human skin mast cells. (A) CXCR1-labeling is mainly present on narrow surface folds (arrowheads). (B) CXCR2-labeling was mainly restricted to mast cell specific granules (arrowheads) and the nucleus. Bars: 0.5 μm.

Chemokines and mast cell secretion

Many well-known chemotactic stimuli induce also a potent secretory response in their target cells (Tab. 2). Surprisingly, although they induced an increase in cytosolic free calcium, none of the CC chemokines studied until now caused release of histamine, tryptase or PGD_2 from human skin mast cells over a wide range of concentrations tested, although basophils did so [31]. Priming of the cells with anti-IgE also failed to change their responsiveness to these mediators [31]. IL-8, MGSA and NAP-2 were also unable to induce release of histamine, LTC_4, tryptase and IL-8 from HMC-1 cells (our own unpublished data). Other groups failed similarly to induce activation of human lung mast cells by RANTES or MCP-1 [32] or to elicit or boost histamine release from intact human skin by microdialysis after perfusion with RANTES, MCP-1 and MIP-1α [33].

In contrast to these negative findings in humans, mast cells from other species selectively exhibit a secretory response to chemokines. Thus, mouse peritoneal mast cells were activated by MIP-1α, but not by MCP-1, -2 and -3 [34, 35]. In another study, MCP-1 caused on the other hand both histamine and serotonin release from rat peritoneal mast cells in a time- and dose-dependent fashion, and it induced his-

Table 2 - Functional response of human mast cells to different chemokines

	Chemotaxis	Secretion	Priming
CXC chemokines			
IL-8	+	−	
MGSA	+	−	
NAP-2	+	−	
PF4	+°		
CC chemokines			
MIP-1α	−*	−*	−*
MIP-1β	−	−	−
MCP-1	−*	−*	−**
MCP-2	−		−
MCP-3	−		−
RANTES	+	−	−

° observed only with murine mast cells
* positive also in murine mast cells
** positive in murine mast cells with IL-3, but not with anti-IgE or compound 48/80

tidine decarboxylase mRNA under these same conditions [36]. The same authors also observed aggregation of mast cells in the presence of MCP-1 by electron microscopy [36], suggesting an enhanced adhesion molecule expression and thus potentially improved immune functions of the cells [37]. Priming of the cells for an enhanced responsiveness to MCP-1 was only observed with IL-3 and not with anti-IgE or compound 48/80 [36]. MCP-1 and MIP-1α have also been shown to cause *in vivo* histamine release from murine skin [38].

Taken together, these data provide a further line of evidence for the heterogeneity of mast cells regarding both species and organ distribution. The mechanisms determining this diversity are unclear. At least in the case of IL-8 and human mast cells, receptor defects as well as calcium mobilization cannot account for the failure of the cells to mount a secretory response.

Biological and pathological significance

The data available until now are at most fragmentary and accordingly provide only an incomplete picture regarding the significance of mast cell chemokine secretion and responsiveness under normal and pathological conditions. They leave however no doubt that mast cells can potentially contribute to the influx of inflammatory cells into the tissue by releasing IL-8 and other chemokines. The production of chemokines by these cells and by resident skin cells like fibroblasts and keratinocytes might in turn induce the influx of mast cells to sites of inflammation, explaining the increase of mast cells, e.g. in tissue of patients with urticaria [2] and diverse other diseases [1].

The potential significance of the ability of mast cells to produce and respond to IL-8 remains enigmatic since cell migration occurs only when a gradient of mediators is established which is not given when the cell itself is the source of the mediator, and human mast cells have until now escaped any attempts to induce functional alterations in response to IL-8 other than chemotaxis. Possibly, since non-gradient exposure to mediators induces immobilization or deactivation of cells, mast cell-derived IL-8 might serve as a negative signal for the inflammatory reaction, also in view of the high level IL-8 secretion from mast cells many hours after initiation of stimulation (see Fig. 1), and it might serve to keep the cells quiescent under physiological conditions.

This idea has in fact been considered by others who observed an increase of IL-8 in allergic patients responding well to immunotherapy, with an associated decrease of several CC chemokines [39]. The authors interpret these findings in view of the ability of IL-8 to act as an inhibitor of histamine release in, for example, basophils whereas CC chemokines like MCP-1, RANTES and MIP-1α have the reverse effect. Unfortunately, no support for this hypothesis by, for example, an examination of the patients' mast cells has been provided until now. From the data summarized here regarding human mast cell histamine release in response to C-C chemokines, this attractive theory cannot be upheld. Further studies will hopefully soon help to lift the veil on the physiopathological significance of human mast cell-derived chemokines.

Acknowledgement

Supported by grant Mo 462/2-2 from the German Research Foundation (DFG).

References

1   Weber S, Krüger-Krasagakes S, Grabbe J, Zuberbier T, Czarnetzki BM (1995) Mast cells. *Int J Dermatol* 34: 1–10

2   Haas N, Toppe E, Henz BM (1998) Microscopic morphology in different types of urticaria. *Arch Dermatol* 134: 41–46

3   Haas N, Motel K, Czarnetzki BM (1995) Comparative immunoreactivity of the eosinophil constituents MBP and ECP in different types of urticaria. *Arch Dermatol Res* 287: 180–185

4   Czarnetzki BM (1987) Mechanisms and mediators in urticaria. *Sem Dermatol* 6:272–285

5   Rosenbach T, Grabbe J, Möller A, Schwanitz HJ, Czarnetzki BM (1985) Generation of leukotrienes from normal epidermis and their demonstration in cutaneous disease. *Br J Dermatol* (Suppl 28) 113: 157–167

6   Wassermann SI, Goetzl EJ, Austen KF (1974) Preformed eosinophil chemotactic factor of anaphylaxis (ECF-A). *J Immunol* 112: 351–358

7   Czarnetzki BM, König W Lichtenstein LM (1976) Antigen-induced eosinophil chemotactic factor (ECF) release by human leukocytes. *Inflammation* 1: 201–215

8   Wassermann SI, Soter NA, Center DM, Austen KF (1977) Cold urticaria. Recognition and characterisation of a neutrophil chemotactic factor which appears in serum during cold challenge. *J Clin Invest* 60: 189–196.

9   Plaut M, Pierce JH, Watson CJ, Hanley-Hyde J, Nordan RP, Paul WE (1989) Mast cell lines produce lymphokines in response to cross-linkage of FcεRI or to calcium ionophores. *Nature* 339: 64–67

10 Möller A, Lippert U, Leßmann D, Kolde G, Hamann K, Welker P, Schadendorf D, Grabbe J, Rosenbach T, Luger T, Czarnetzki BM (1993) Human mast cells produce IL-8. *J Immunol* 151: 3261–66

11 Möller A, Grabbe J, Czarnetzki BM (1991) Mast cells and their mediators in immediate and delayed immune reactions. *Skin Pharmacol* 4 (suppl 1): 56–63

12 Nilsson G, Blom T, Kusche-Gullberg M, Kjellen L, Butterfield JH, Sundström C, Nilsson K, Hellman L (1994) Phenotypic characterization of the human mast-cell line HMC-1. *Scand J Immunol* 39: 489–498

13 Hamann K, Grabbe J, Welker P, Haas N, Algermissen B, Czarnetzki BM (1994) Pheno-
    typic evaluation of cultured human mast and basophilic cells and of normal human skin
    mast cells. *Arch Dermatol Res* 286: 380–385

14 Möller A, Henz BM, Grützkau A, Lippert U, Schwarz T, Aragane Y, Krüger-Krasagakes
    S (1998) Comparative cytokine gene expression, regulation and release by human mast
    cells. *Immunology* 93: 289–295

15 Buckley MG, Williams CMM, Thompson J, Pryor P, Ray P, Butterfield JH, Coleman JW
    (1995) IL-4 enhances IL-3 and IL-8 gene expression in a human leukemic mast cell line.
    Immunology 84: 410–415

16 Lippert U, Krüger-Krasagakes S, Möller A, Kiessling U, Czarnetzki BM (1995) Pharma-
    cological modulation of IL-6 and IL-8 secretion by the H1-antagonist descarboethoxy-
    loratadine and dexamethasone from human mast and basophilic cell lines. *Exp Derma-
    tol* 4: 272–276

17 Grützkau A, Krüger-Krasagakes S, Kögel H, Möller A, Lippert U, Henz BM (1997).
    Detection of intracellular interleukin-8 in the human mast cell line-1: Using flow
    cytometry as a guide for immunoelectron microscopy. *J Histochem Cytochem* 45:
    935–945

18 Selvan RS, Butterfield JH, Krangel MS (1994) Expression of multiple chemokine genes
    by a human mast cell leukemia. *J Biol Chem* 269: 13893–13898

19 Safari MN, Garcia-Zepeda EA, MacLean JA, Charo IF, Luster AD (1997) Murine
    monocyte chemoattractant protein (MCP)-5: A novel CC chemokine that is a structur-
    al and functional homologue of human MCP-1. *J Exp Med* 185: 99–109

20 Kulmburg PA, Huber NE, Scheer BJ, Wrann M, Baumruker T (1992) Immunoglobulin
    E plus antigen challenge induces a novel intercrine/chemokine in mouse mast cells. *J Exp
    Med* 176: 1773–1778

21 Jarmin DI, Kulmburg PA, Huber NE, Baumann G, Prieschl-Strassmayr EE, Baumruker
    T (1994) A transcription factor with AP3-like binding specificity mediates gene regula-
    tion after allergic triggering with IgE and Ag in mouse mast cells. *J Immunol* 153:
    5720–5729

22 Prieschl EE, Pendl GG, Harrer NE, Baumruker T (1995) p21ras links FcRI to NF-AT
    family member in mast cells. *J Immunol* 155: 4963–4970

23 Noso N, Krüger-Krasagakes S, Czarnetzki BM, Schröder JM (1995) Analysis of HMC-
    1 mast cell-line derived eosinophil attractants. J Invest Dermatol 105: 717

24 Rumsaeng V, Vliagoftis H, Oh CK, Metcalfe DD (1997) Lymphotactin gene expression
    in mast cells following Fcε receptor I aggregation. *J Immunol* 158: 1353–1360

25 Rot A (1992) Binding of neutrophil attractant/activation protein-1 (interleukin 8) to res-
    ident dermal cells. *Cytokine* 4: 347–352

26 Premack BA, Schall TJ (1996) Chemokine receptors: Gateway to inflammation and
    infection. *Nature Medicine* 2: 1174–1178

27 Lippert U, Artuc M, Grützkau A, Schadendorf D, Möller A, Czarnetzki BM, Krüger-
    Krasagakes S (1995) Expression and functional activity of the IL-8 receptor in the
    human mast cell line HMC-1. *J Invest Dermatol* 105: 717

28 Lippert U, Artuc M, Grützkau A, Möller A, Kenderessy-Szabo A, Schadendorf D, Nor-gauer J, Hartmann K, Zuberbier T, Schweizer-Stenner R et al (1998) Expression and functional activity of the IL-8 receptor type CXCR1 and CXCR2 on human mast cells. *J Immunol; in press*

29 Nilsson G, Butterfield JH, Nilsson K, Siegbahn A (1994) Stem cell factor is a chemo-tactic factor for human mast cells. *J Immunol* 153: 3717–3723

30 Taub D, Dastych J, Inamura N, Upton J, Kelvin D, Metcalfe D, Oppenheim J (1995) Bone marrow-derived murine mast cells migrate, but do not degranulate, in response to chemokines. *J Immunol* 154: 2393–2402

31 Hartmann K, Beiglböck F, Czarnetzki BM, Zuberbier T (1995) Effect of CC chemokines on mediator release from human skin mast cells and basophils. *Int Arch Allergy Immunol* 108: 224–230

32 Takaishi T, Morita Y, Hirai K, Yamaguchi M, Ohta K, Noda E, Morita T, Ito K, Miyamoto T (1994) Effect of cytokines on mediator release from human dispersed lung mast cells. *Allergy* 49: 837–842

33 Petersen LJ, Brasso K. Pryds M, Skov PS (1996) Histamine release in intact human skin by monocyte chemoattractant factor-1α, RANTES, macrophage inflammatory protein-1, stem cell factor, anti-IgE, and codeine as determined by an *ex vivo* skin microdialysis technique. *J Allergy Clin Immunol* 98: 790–796

34 Alam R, Forsythe P, Stafford S, Henrich J, Bravo R, Proost P, van Damme J (1994) Monocyte chemotactic protein-2, monocyte chemotactic protein-3, and fibroblast-induced cytokine. Three new chemokines induce chemotaxis and activation of baso-phils. *J Immunol* 153: 3155–3159

35 Alam R, Forsythe P, Stafford S, Lett-Brown MA, Grant JA (1992) Macrophage inflam-matory protein-1 activates basophils and mast cells. *J Exp Med* 176: 781–786

36 Conti P, Boucher W, Letourneau R, Feliciani C, Reale M, Barbacane RC, Vlagopoulos P, Bruneau G, Thibault J, Theoharides TC (1995) Monocyte chemotactic protein-1 pro-vokes mast cell aggregation and ³[H]5HT release. *Immunology* 86: 434–440

37 Weber S, Ruh B, Dippel E, Czarnetzki BM (1994) Monoclonal antibodies to leukosialin (CD 43) induce homotypic aggregation of the human mast cell line HMC-1. Character-ization of leucosialin on HMC-1 cells. *Immunology* 82: 638–644

38 Alam R, Kumar D, Anderson-Walters D, Forsythe P (1994) Macrophage inflammatory protein-1α and monocyte chemoattractant peptide-1 elicit immediate and late cutaneous reactions and activate murine mast cells *in vivo*. *J Immunol* 152: 1298–1303

39 Hsieh K-H, Chou CC, Chiang BL (1996) Immunotherapy suppresses the production of monocyte chemotactic and activating factors and augments the production of IL-8 in children with asthma. *J Allergy Clin Immunol* 98: 580–587

Chemokines and eosinophils

Jens-M. Schröder

Department of Dermatology, University of Kiel, Schittenhelmstr. 7, D-24105 Kiel, Germany

Introduction

Eosinophils (Eos) are recognized as proinflammatory cells implicated in protection against parasitic infection [1] and likely play a major role in allergic diseases such as bronchial asthma, and a number of dermatologic diseases including atopic dermatitis [2–4]. They can release from their granules several distinctive cationic proteins that have the potential to cause local tissue damage and dysfunction seen in many eosinophilic inflammatory skin diseases [1]. Specific cytoplasmic granules contain a unique crystalloid core composed of major basic protein (MBP), which is responsible for the cardinal tinctorial properties of the eosinophil [1]. In addition three other distinct cationic proteins, eosinophil-derived neurotoxin (EDN), eosinophil cationic protein (ECP), and eosinophil peroxidase (EPO), which exert a range of biological effects on host cells and microbial targets, have been found in eosinophils [1].

Interestingly, intradermal injection of ECP results in strong pruritus, which is not inhibitable by antihistaminic agents and which is characteristic for some eosinophilic skin diseases such as atopy [5], and therefore points towards an important role of Eos in particular inflammatory skin diseases.

Eosinophil-chemotactic mediators

Recruitment of eosinophils into inflammatory sites involves a series of events including increase of the number of circulating cells, adhesion to endothelial cells, diapedesis and subsequent tissue infiltration. The number of circulating Eos will be elevated by increased release of Eos from the bone marrow. Mediators which are involved in this process are the hemopoietins IL-3 [6], GMCSF [7] and, more selective for Eos, IL-5 [8, 9]. In addition these growth factors are potent activators and priming agents for Eos, acting at subnanomolar concentrations [9].

Chemokines and Skin, edited by E. Kownatzki and J. Norgauer

Table 1 - Human eosinophil attractants

Attractant	Activity for Eos**	Activity for other leukocytes
C5a	+++++	Neu, Mo
FMLP	++	Neu, Mo
PAF	+++++	Neu, (Mo)
LTB$_4$	+	Neu, Mo
5-oxo ETE*	+++++	Neu

Neu = neutrophils, Mo = monocytes

* 5-oxo-eicosatetraenoic acid

** Relative efficacy (percentage of input migrating cells) in in vitro experiments using the Boyden chamber system (N. Noso and J.-M. Schröder, unpublished data).

Adhesion of Eos to the luminal side of postcapillary venules seems to be achieved by binding via activation of Eo-integrins and binding to endothelial cell VCAM and integrins [10]. It has been reported that the Eo-integrin VLA-4 possesses a selectivity for Eos and thus represents a candidate mediator for Eo-selective tissue infiltration [11]. This process seems to be controlled by IL-4, which induces selective endothelium driven transmigration of Eos from allergic individuals [12].

After diapedesis through endothelium of postcapillary venules Eos are believed to migrate into the skin tissue via a gradient of chemotactic factors generated within the tissue.

Some well characterized neutrophil- and monocyte-attractants have been reported to be Eo-attractants as well (Tab. 1). The complement split product C5a represents one of the most potent and efficient Eo-chemotaxins [13]. Platelet-activating factor (PAF) has been reported to be a very effective chemotaxin for human Eos [14]. Indeed, when compared with other pan-leukotactic mediators (except C5a) it was seen to express the highest chemotactic index (percentage of migrating cells) in vitro [13].

Although leukotriene B$_4$ (LTB$_4$) induces some locomotory responses in human Eos [15], it is much more effective in guinea pig Eos. A recently discovered family of novel eicosanoids – 5-oxo-eicosanoids – [16] are as effective as PAF as Eo-attractant in vitro. Its relevance in the in vivo accumulation of Eos at present is rather speculative.

Eosinophil-selective proteinaceous chemotaxins

In previous studies it has been suggested that products of immediate type (anaphy-lactic) reactions contain eosinophil selective attractants. Two tetrapeptides, Val-Gly-Ser-Glu and Ala-Gly-Ser-Glu, were extracted from resected human lung and were believed to comprise part of the Eo-chemotactic activity contained in challenged lung supernatants [17].

However, these peptides were found to be inactive in attracting Eos *in vitro* in numerous laboratories including our own (data not shown).

The effects of hemopoietins such as IL-5 on Eo-production in the bone marrow [18] later led to the hypothesis that these growth factors activate eosinophils and induce locomotory responses. Indeed, in recent investigations it has been shown that rhIL-5 [9, 19], GMCSF [20] and IL-3 [6] stimulate *in vitro* migratory responses in Eos and not in neutrophils and monocytes. Furthermore, when GMCSF was inject-ed subcutaneously, Eos represented – apart from lymphocytes – the most prominent cellular infiltrate cell type [21]. Specificity of IL-5 for Eos originally led to over-estimation of IL-5 as Eo-attractant. *In vivo* detectable levels of IL-5 rarely induce Eo-chemotaxis *in vitro*.

Apart from Eo-hemopoietins it has been reported that CD4-binding ligands such as "lymphocyte chemoattractant Factor, LCF," now termed IL-16 [22], which is released by histamin-stimulated T-lymphocytes, are very potent and efficient Eo-chemotaxins. So far there is no published information whether IL-16 is generated in inflamed skin and whether cells other than T-lymphocytes are also capable to release this cytokine.

Eosinophil-chemotactic chemokines

Apart from the Eo-attractants described above, more recently a family of leukocyte-form and sub-type-selective chemotactic cytokines, now termed chemokines, has been detected, members of which have preferential chemotactic properties for neu-trophils, monocytes, lymphocytes and – as recently shown – also Eos. Table 2 sum-marizes the origin and function of Eo-activating chemokines. As the first Eo-chemo-tactic chemokine the CC-chemokine RANTES (acronym for *r*egulated *a*nd *n*ormal *T*-lymphocyte *e*xpressed and presumably *s*ecreted) has been discovered [23]. RANTES was seen to be released from thrombin-stimulated platelets [23]. Interest-ingly, platelets were the first natural cellular source reported of biologically active RANTES. Other studies have shown that recombinant RANTES is as active as the natural form [24, 25].

The Eo-chemotactic index (percentage of input migrating Eos) of RANTES var-ied from donor to donor [26]. This unexpected phenomenon might be explained by the presence of Eos, which did not respond to RANTES [27] possibly by reduced receptor densities.

Table 2 - Origin and function of Eo-activating chemokines

Chemokine	species	structural subfamily	receptor	major cellular origin[4]	major target cell	major function in vitro	major function in vivo
RANTES	h[1]	CC	CCR1, CCR5, CCR3	Plts, T Ly, Fib	T Ly, Mo, Eo	Mo and Eo Chemoattr.	Mo-recruitment? memory T cell recruitment? in TH1 reactions?
MIP-1	h	CC	CCR1	T Ly	T Ly (Eo)	?	stem cell proliferation inhibitor?
MCP-2	h	CC	CCR2, CCR5	Fib	Mo, T Ly (Eo)	Mo-chemoattr.	?
MCP-3	h	CC	CCR5, CCR3	?	Mo, Eo	Mo, Eo-chemoattr.	?
MCP-4	h	CC	CCR3, CCR5	?	Mo, T Ly Eo	Eo-chemoattr.	?
MARC	m	CC	?	Mastc.	?	?	?
Eotaxin	gp[2]	CC	?	?	Eo	specific Eo chemoattr.	Eo-recruitment in allergy
Eotaxin	m[3]	CC	?	?	Eo	specific Eo chemoattr.	Eo-recruitment in allergy
Eotaxin	h	CC	CCR3	Fib	Eo, TH2-Ly	specific Eo and TH2 chemoattr.	Eo and Th2-Ly tissue recruitment?
Eotaxin 2	h	CC	CCR3	?	Eo	specific Eo chemoattr.	?
IL-8	h	CXC	CXCR1, CXCR2	Mo, End, Fib, Ker	Neu, (Eo) (T Ly)	Neu-chemoattr.	Neu recruitment

[1] human, [2] guinea pig, [3] mouse, [4] Plts = platelets, T Ly = T lymphocytes, Fib = fibroblasts, Mo = monocytes, Mastc = mast cells, End = endothelial cells, Ker = keratinocytes, Eo = Eosinophils, Neu = neutrophil

Skin cells can produce RANTES: Cultivated dermal fibroblasts were shown to be capable of expressing RANTES mRNA and release immunoreactive RANTES upon stimulation with TNF-α, IL-1α and IL-1β [28]. The production of RANTES by dermal fibroblasts might be important for Eo-tissue infiltration, which usually occurs only in the dermis and not epidermis.

Dermal fibroblast-derived RANTES is biologically active. Biochemical purification identified it as the 66-residue form of RANTES [29], which was found to be as active as the platelet-derived 68-residue form [23]. The amounts of biologically active RANTES produced by cultivated dermal fibroblasts were extremely high. More than 1 µg per 10^6 cells was secreted upon TNF-α-stimulation [29]. In contrast to these cells, cultivated endothelial cells produced very low amounts (~10 ng per 10^6 cells) of RANTES and only when stimulated with IFNγ plus TNFα, according to a previous study [30]. Although keratinocyte cell lines expressed RANTES mRNA and secreted immunoreactive RANTES, as yet it is not clear whether normal keratinocytes are capable of producing biologically active RANTES and thus could be an important cellular source of RANTES in cutaneous inflammation.

In vitro effects of RANTES on eosinophils include chemotactic activity, trans-endothelial migration, release of ECP and induction of the production of reactive oxygen species [25, 31]. Whereas RANTES also has been reported to increase the expression of the cell surface adhesion molecule Mac-1 (CD11b/CD18) [25], it failed to induce VLA-4.

Evidence for an *in vivo* role of RANTES as an eosinophil chemoattractant was presented by a study showing that intradermal injection of RANTES into dogs leads to an inflammatory infiltrate mainly consisting of eosinophils and monocytes [32]. In humans intradermal injection of RANTES into normal, non-atopic volunteers resulted in endothelial swelling and neutrophil accumulation within postcapillary venules. Interestingly, signs of Eo-accumulation or infiltration could not be observed [33].

Monocyte chemotactic proteins (MCPs)

Apart from the CC chemokines MIP-1α and RANTES also some of the monocyte chemotactic proteins (MCPs), which share considerable sequence similarity with each other (60–71%), have been reported to elicit functional responses in eosinophils – apart from their major activity in monocytes (Tab. 3).

Whereas MCP-1 does not activate Eos, MCP-2 is a weak attractant for human Eos [34, 35]. Efficacy (percentage of input migrating cells) is less than that seen with RANTES. Synthetic MCP-2 [35] showed similar Eo-chemotactic properties *in vitro* as seen for natural material [34].

Only limited data exist on *in vitro* and *in vivo* regulation of these chemokines. Although the cDNA cloning of MCP-2 (synonym with HC-14) has been reported [36] neither cDNA nor genomic sequences were available.

Table 3 - Human eosinophil-activating chemokines

Chemokine	Activity for Eos	Activity for other leukocytes
RANTES	+++	memory T Ly, Mo, Bas
MCP-2	++	Mo, T Ly, Bas
MCP-3	+++	Mo, Bas, T Ly
MCP-4	+++	Mo, Bas, T Ly
Eotaxin	++++	no
Eotaxin 2	+++	?

T Ly = T lymphocytes, Mo = monocytes, Bas = basophils

MCP-2 was originally identified as a low level secreted monocyte chemoattractant produced by some tumor cell lines and fibroblast cell lines, when these were stimulated with IL-1, interferon-γ, mitogens, double-stranded RNA, and viruses [37].

MCP-3 is another monocyte- and eosinophil-chemotactic CC-chemokine, that attracted attention as a possible mediator of allergic inflammation due to similarity to the murine C-C chemokine MARC, which is expressed upon allergic stimulation (IgE plus allergen) in a murine mast cell line [38].

MCP-3 *in vitro* shows strong Eo-chemotactic activity [34, 39]. MCP-3 mRNA is expressed in a number of tumor cells and cell lines upon stimulation with IL-1, interferon-α, mitogens, inferferon-γ, double strand RNA and viruses [37]. After discovery of MCP-3 protein, which was found in minute amounts as monocyte-chemotaxin in osteosarcoma cell supernatants [38], there is no published report that normal cells are producing bioactive MCP-3 protein. This is surprising because a number of cells including normal dermal fibroblasts (unpublished results) showed strong MCP-3 mRNA expression upon stimulation with IL-1β or interferon-α.

It needs to be clarified whether additional posttranscriptional regulatory mechanisms do exist for MCP-3 or whether preformed cell-stored material is not released or only released under as yet unknown conditions. Thus MCP-3 is an additional candidate Eo-chemotactic chemokine of putative importance in skin Eo-infiltration.

Recent cloning of a new cDNA revealed a predicted protein with marked sequence similarities to MCPs that subsequently was termed MCP-4 [39].

MCP-4 is an efficient chemotaxin for human Eos that is probably more potent than MCP-3. It also activates monocytes and lymphocytes [39].

Information about cellular sources of MCP-4 and conditions of its gene expression and/or protein release is still lacking.

Eotaxins

The striking accumulation of eosinophils in certain tissues suggest that there may be factors that are specific for eosinophils. In sensitized guinea pigs after allergen challenge in the lung an Eo-specific CC-chemokine was identified that subsequently was termed eotaxin [40]. Eotaxin is highly potent in guinea pigs, inducing substantial eosinophil accumulation at a 1-2 pmol dose in the skin [40]. More recent investigations showed that also in mice an eotaxin exists [41]. Based on partial mouse or guinea pig eotaxin cDNA probes recently the human eotaxin gene was cloned [42–44].

Human eotaxin is a strong chemoattractant for normal human Eos, but is not chemotactic for neutrophils and lymphocytes, and only at very high concentration modestly chemotactic for monocytes [42–44].

When injected intradermally into adult rhesus monkeys at doses of 10 pmol eosinophils were recruited, which histologically were seen clustered throughout the dermal collagen bundles [42].

Northern blot analyses revealed a strong constitutive eotaxin gene expression in the small intestine, colon and heart [42]. Eotaxin mRNA was seen in cultured human cells upon stimulation: endothelial cells express eotaxin mRNA upon stimulation with TNF-α, IL-1α, IFNγ plus TNFα, but not IL-4 [43].

Similarly respiratory epithelial cells express eotaxin mRNA upon stimulation with IFNγ plus TNF-α [43]. In another study, Lilly and coworkers [45] demonstrated eotaxin mRNA expression in airway epithelial cells after stimulation with IL-1β or TNF-α, which was enhanced by adding IFNγ. Using a specific ELISA immunoreactive eotaxin was seen to be released in amounts of a few pg per 10^6 cells with the same stimuli, thus insufficient concentrations are known to elicit strong eosinophil responses *in vitro*.

When we looked for the production of Eo-specific cytokines by skin cells we could identify bioactive eotaxin in supernatants of dermal fibroblasts stimulated for at least 3 days with TNF-α (N. Noso and J.-M. Schröder, unpublished results). Surprisingly three cDNA variants of eotaxin have been identified indicating possible gene polymorphism [46]. In recent investigations we found that the TH2 cytokine IL-4 is a potent and rapid (within hours) inducer of eotaxin (M. Mochizuki, J. Bartels and J.-M. Schröder, unpublished results).

The natural eotaxin produced via IL-4 induction showed slightly different biochemical properties when compared with that form secreted after TNF-α-stimulation (N. Noso and J.-M. Schröder, unpublished results). Interestingly, costimulation of dermal fibroblasts with IL-4 and TNF-α induced a strong production (10–20 fold increase) of three biochemically and biologically different natural forms of eotaxin (M. Mochizuki, J. Bartels and J.-M. Schröder, unpublished results).

Whereas dermal fibroblasts appear to be a rich cellular source of eotaxin, as yet our experiments failed to detect bioactive eotaxin in supernatants of stimulated endothelial cells, keratinocytes, mononuclear phagocytes and lymphocytes (M. Mochizuki, J. Bartels and J.-M. Schröder, unpublished results).

Recently another novel CC-chemokine termed eotaxin-2 has been discovered [47]. Eotaxin-2 is a highly potent, efficient and Eo-selective chemotaxin, however, it is nearly one order of magnitude less potent than eotaxin [47].

Due to the very recent discovery, cellular sources, conditions of its production and thus its role in cutaneous inflammation is unknown.

Activation of Eo-functions via chemokine receptors

Apart from activating migratory responses, the chemokines RANTES, MIP-1α, MCP-2, MCP-3, MCP-4, eotaxin as well as eotaxin-2 elicit a number of other Eo-functions.

These chemokines also activate the release of reactive oxygen species (ROS) by Eos: rEotaxin elicited similar responses as C5a, one of the most efficient agents [48], whereas MCP-3 and RANTES [27] were found to be less effective.

MIP-1α did not activate ROS release [24] but elicited a rise of $[Ca^{2+}]_i$ in human Eos. Moreover IL-8, RANTES, MIP 1α, MCP-3 and eotaxin have been reported to induce actin polymerization in IL-5 primed cells [49].

When Eos were pretreated with cytochalasin B RANTES as well as MIP-1α induced the release of Eosinophil cationic protein (ECP) at 10^{-8}–10^{-7} M concentrations [24]. Eotaxin was found to induce ECP release at similar concentrations. In contrast to studies with C5a neither RANTES nor MIP-1α were capable to induce the generation of LTC$_4$ [24].

Chemokines are known to bind to and signal through G-protein coupled receptors with seven transmembrane spanning domains. Whereas various chemokine receptors are expressed on leukocytes (for review see [50]), the array of chemokines described above, which all activate Eos, suggested a complex pattern of receptor expression on Eos. CCR1, the MIP-1α/RANTES receptor, was initially considered as a possible Eo receptor for CC-chemokines [51], but desensitization experiments ($[Ca^{2+}]_i$ and chemotaxis) and ligand binding studies implicated the existence of a distinct Eo-receptor.

CCR3, the eotaxin receptor, was subsequently identified as major CC chemokine receptor on eosinophils [42, 44]. When transfected into a cell line, CCR3 bound eotaxin, RANTES and MCP-3, but not MIP-1α. Whether Eos bear CCR1, CCR2, CCR4 and CCR5 is still unclear, as is the receptor on eosinophils used by MCP-4 and MCP-2. Functional effects of all of the efficacious chemokines for eosinophils – eotaxin, RANTES, MCP-2, MCP-3, or MCP-4 – could be blocked completely with a specific anti CCR3 mAb [52], indicating that CCR3 represents the principal receptor for Eo responses to chemokines and questions an essential role for CCR1, CCR2, CCR4, or CCR5.

Donor to donor variation in eosinophil responses to RANTES and other Eo-activating CC-chemokines might be explained by receptor downregulation or absence in subpopulations [53]. Indeed, some of the Eos stimulated with RANTES did not show any signs of activation [27]. It has been demonstrated that IL-8, which does not stimulate Eos of normal donors [54], was an attractant for Eos of atopic and asthmatic patients [49, 55] and attracted normal Eos when primed *in vitro* with IL-5.

Using mAbs against the IL-8 receptors CXCR1 and CXCR2, immunoreactive IL-8 receptors were undetectable on Eos from normal individuals [52]. 5–7 days of culture *in vitro* with IL-3, CXCR2 and to a lesser degree CXCR1 were detectable on the surface of Eos, whereas CCR3 was not affected [52]. These effects paralleled the ability of Eos to migrate to IL-8 [53]. The relevance of IL-8 receptors on primed or activated Eos is uncertain.

Eosinophils can produce chemokines

A number of studies have shown that eosinophils can act as a cellular source of various cytokines and mediators [56]. IL-8 is secreted by Eos, when stimulated with a Ca^{2+}-ionophore [57]. More recently it was demonsrated that significant amounts of IL-8 were released in response to C5a or FMLP, but only when Eos were pretreated with cytochalasin B [58].

Eo-activating chemokines, such as RANTES and MIP-1α, failed to generate IL-8 in Eos [58]. Apart from IL-8 it was demonstrated that Eos express MIP-1α mRNA, when isolated from hypereosinophilic patients but not from normal subjects [59].

MCP-1 protein release was strongly stimulated with C5a and to a lesser extent with FMLP, when Eos were pretreated with cytochalasin B [60]. Interestingly IL-5 pretreatment of Eos increased C5a-dependent MCP-1 production nearly threefold [60].

Eo-activating chemokines in eosinophilic diseases

At present, only few data are available that directly document the involvement of chemokines in these diseases. In a recent study it was shown that skin biopsies of atopic donors challenged with allergens contained cells that expressed mRNA for RANTES and MCP-3. But only MCP-3 mRNA paralleled the kinetics of Eo-infiltration [61]. Data showing that MCP-3 protein is formed and released are lacking.

The different kinetics of RANTES mRNA and MCP-3 mRNA expression led to the hypothesis that RANTES may have more relevance to the later accumulation of

T cells and macrophages [61], because it is known to be also a memory T cell- and macrophage-activating chemokine [62].

In order to investigate the participation of Eo-chemotactic chemokines in eosinophilic dermatoses, we recently identified a single peak of Eo-chemotactic activity that copurified with immunoreactive RANTES in lesional scales of patients with drug reactions [53].

Under similar conditions in scales of atopic dermatitis patients no Eo-chemotactic activity but immunoreactive RANTES was detected [53]. Thus it is possible that RANTES may not represent the major Eo attractant in allergic inflammation. This hypothesis is further supported by a recent observation that 24 h after allergen challenge of asthmatic patients RANTES was released into the lung, but the rate/kinetics of release did not correlate with Eo infiltration [63]. Instead, Eo-infiltration correlated with the TH_2-cytokine IL-5.

Recent studies on the chemokine production of TH_1 and TH_2-like T lymphocytes surprisingly revealed that RANTES is produced predominantly by TH_1 cells [64], thus supporting the idea that RANTES represents rather a TH_1- than TH_2-cytokine.

An association between TH_2-responses and Eo-tissue infiltration is a well known phenomenon. Thus IL-4 or other TH_2 cytokines might be involved in eosinophil recruitment. This hypothesis is also based on the observation that transgenic mice expressing IL-4 in the lung show eosinophilic lung inflammation [65], and in IL-4-deficient mice tissue eosinophilia is inhibited upon *onchocerca volvulus* mediated corneal inflammation [66] and upon allergen-induced airway inflammation [67].

We investigated whether the TH_2 cytokine IL-4 induced the production of Eo-attractants in dermal fibroblasts. To our surprise, there was strong and Eo-specific chemotactic activity, which could be attributed to eotaxin. Interestingly, IL-4 stimulated dermal fibroblasts to produce eotaxin and secrete a biologically active protein [68]. The release was strongly increased upon stimulation with TNF-α. It is attractive to speculate that this mechanism is responsible for the association between TH_2 cytokines and selective Eo-accumulation in the dermis seen in helminth parasite infections and in atopic and allergic skin diseases [69]. Furthermore, the release of preformed IL-4 together with TNF-α from mast cells [70] might result in strong eotaxin release from dermal fibroblasts *in vivo* – although so far this has not been shown.

Outlook

The demonstration that Eos appear to play an important role as effector cells in parasitic helminth infection and allergic and atopic skin diseases has stimulated many researchers to investigate the mechanisms by which these cells migrate into the inflammatory site. The discovery of the chemokines and the finding that some of them are potent Eo-chemoattractants identified them as potential mediators of allergic inflammation. Considerable evidence indicates important roles for CC chemokines in cutaneous allergic inflammation. The question, however, arises of whether the involved CC chemokines are specific for eosinophilic (allergic) inflammation. For example, RANTES has been seen to be expressed in numerous diseases – apart from allergic inflammation [70]. Eotaxin in mice is not restricted to a TH_2-type response, and eotaxin mRNA is also upregulated by LPS administration, a stimulus that favors neutrophilia rather than eosinophilia [71].

Is there a species specific response? For example MIP-1α is a strong Eo-attractant in mice, however, in humans it is a poor stimulus. Therefore, information that comes from animal experiments may not be directly applicable to humans.

Recently it was predicted that the total number of chemokines – when finally known – could exceed 100 [71], leading to the possibility that also novel Eo-attracting chemokines are among them.

Currently, eotaxin and CCR 3 show promise as targets for therapeutic intervention in eosinophilic dermatoses. Inhibition of Eo-tissue infiltration by inhibiting either production of Eo-specific chemokines and/or receptor binding is an attractive working hypothesis for therapeutic intervention. So far, however, strong evidence for the decisive role of a particular chemokine in the pathophysiology of eosinophilic inflammation is lacking. The majority of data is based upon mRNA expression and in some cases also upon immunoreactive protein expression. Only a few studies show the release of bioactive cytokines. Thus the redundancy of the many different Eo-chemotactic CC chemokines discovered so far might not be as confusing as expected, because only a few will be expressed as bioactive proteins, possibly only under particular conditions in tissue cells.

Future studies will have to find out these conditions, which will help to understand the tissue-site selectivity of cell infiltration, that is so characteristic for eosinophils.

Acknowledgement

This work was supported by Deutsche Forschungsgemeinschaft, grant Ch 38/7-2.

References

1   Weller PF (1994) Eosinophils: structure and functions. *Curr Opinion in Immunol* 6: 85–90
2   Leiferman KM, Ackerman SJ, Sampson HA, Peters MS, Gleich GJ (1995) Dermal deposition of eosinophil-granule major basic protein in atopic dermatitis: comparison with onchocerciasis. *N Engl J Med* 313: 282–285

3   Peters MS, Schroeter AL, Kephart GM, Gleich GJ (1983) Localization of eosinophil granule major basic protein in chronic urticaria. *J Invest Dermatol* 81: 39–43

4   Leiferman KM, Fujisawa T, Gray BH, Gleich GJ (1990) Extracellular deposition of eosinophil and neutrophil granule proteins in the IgE-mediated cutaneous late phase reaction. *Lab Invest* 62: 579–589

5   Gleich GJ, Adolphson CR (1986) The eosinophilic leukocyte: structure and function. *Adv Immunol* 39: 177–253

6   Lopez AF, To LB, Yang Y-C, Gamble JR, Shannon MF, Burms GF, Dyson PG, Juttner CA, Clark S, Vadas MA (1987) Stimulation of proliferation, differentiation, and function of human cells by primate interleukin 3. *Proc Natl Acad Sci USA* 84: 2761–2765

7   Metcalf D (1985) The granulocyte-macrophage colony stimulating factor. *Science* 229: 16–22

8   Lopez AF, Begley CG, Williamson DF, Warren DJ, Vadas MA, Sanderson CJ (1986) Murine eosinophil differentiation factor. An eosinophil-specific colony-stimulating factor with activity for human cells. *J Exp Med* 163: 1085

9   Lopez AF, Sanderson CJ, Gamble JR, Campbell HD, Young IG, Vadas MA (1988) Recombinant human Interleukin 5 is a selective activator of human eosinophil function. *J Exp Med* 167: 219–224

10   Walsh GM, Mermod J-J, Hartnell A, Kay AB, Wardlaw AJ (1991) Human eosinophil, but not neutrophil, adherence to IL-1-stimulated human umbilical vascular endothelial cells is α4β1 (very late Antigen-4) dependent. *J Immunol* 146: 3419–3423

11   Weg, VB, Williams, TJ, Lobb, RR, Nourshargh, SA (1993) Monoclonal antibody recognizing very late activation antigen 4 inhibits eosinophil accumulation *in vivo*. *J Exp Med* 177: 561–566

12   Moser R, Fehr J, Bruijnzeel PLB (1992) IL-4 controls the selective endothelium-driven transmigration of eosinophils from allergic individuals. *J Immunol* 149: 1432–1438

13   Morita E, Schröder J-M, Christophers E (1989) Differential sensitivities of purified human eosinophils and neutrophils to defined chemotaxins. *Scand J Immunol* 29: 709–716

14   Wardlaw AJ, Moqbel R, Cromwell O, Kay AB (1986) Platelet-activating factor: a potent chemotactic and chemokinetic factor for human eosinophils. *J Clin Invest* 78: 1701–1706

15   Uden AM, Palmblad J, Lindgren JA, Malmsten C (1983) Effects of novel lipoxygenase products on migration of eosinophils and neutrophils *in vitro*. *Int Arch Allergy Appl Immunol* 72: 91–97

16   Schwenk U, Morita E, Engel R, Schröder JM (1992) Identification of 5-oxo-15-hydroxy-6, 8, 11, 13-eicosatetraenoic acid as a novel and potent human eosinophil chemotactic eicosanoid. *J Biol Chem* 267: 12482–12488

17   Goetzl EJ, Austen KF (1975) Purification and synthesis of eosinophilotactic tetrapeptides of human lung: identification as human eosinophil chemotactic factor of anaphylaxis. *Proc Natl Acad Sci USA* 72: 4123

18   Clutterbuck EJ, Sanderson CJ (1988) Human eosinophil hematopoiesis studied *in vitro*

by means of murine eosinophil differentiation factor (IL-5): production of functionally active eosinophils from normal human bone marrow. *Blood* 71: 646–651

19 Wang JM, Rambaldi A, Biondi A, Chen ZG, Sanderson CJ, Mantovani A (1989) Recombinant human interleukin 5 is a selective eosinophil chemoattractant. *Eur J Immunol* 19: 701–708

20 Owen WF, Rothenberg ME, Silberstein DS, Gasson JC, Stevens RL, Austen KF, Soberman RF (1987) Regulation of human eosinophil viability, density and functional activity by granulocyte/macrophage colony-stimulating factor in the presence of 3T3 fibroblasts. *J Exp Med* 166: 129–137

21 Mehregan DR, Franswag AF, Edmonson JH, Leiferman KM (1992) Cutaneous reactions to granulocyte-monocyte colony-stimulating factor. *Arch Dermatol* 128: 1055–1059

22 Rand TH, Cruikshank WW, Center DM, Weller PF (1991) CD4-mediated stimulation of human eosinophils: lymphocyte chemoattractant factor and other CD4-binding ligands elicit eosinophil migration. *J Exp Med* 173: 1521–1528

23 Kameyoshi Y, Dörschner A, Mallet AI, Christophers E, Schröder J-M (1992) Cytokine RANTES released by thrombin-stimulated platelets is a potent attractant for human eosinophils. *J Exp Med* 176: 587–592

24 Rot A, Kriger M, Brunner T, Bischoff SC, Schall TJ, Dahinden CA (1992) RANTES and macrophage inflammatory protein 1α induce the migration and activation of normal human eosinophil granulocytes. *J Exp Med* 176: 1489–1495

25 Alam R, Stafford S, Forsythe P, Harrison R, Faubion D, Lett-Brown MA, Grant IA (1993) RANTES is a chemotactic and activating factor for human eosinophils. *J Immunol* 150: 3442–3447

26 Schröder J-M, Kameyoshi Y, Christophers E (1993) Platelets secrete an eosinophil-chemotactic cytokine which is a member of the CC chemokine family. In: IJD Lindley, J Westwick, S. Kunkel (eds): *The chemokines*. Plenum Press, New York, 119–128

27 Kapp A, Zeck-Kapp G, Czech W, Schöpf E (1994) The chemokine RANTES is more than a chemoattractant: Characterization of its effect on human eosinophil oxidative metabolism and morphology in comparison with IL-5 and GM-CSF. *J Invest Dermatol* 102: 906–914

28 Sticherling M, Küpper M, Koltrowitz F, Bornscheuer E, Kulke R, Klinger M, Wilhelm D, Kameyoshi Y, Christophers E, Schröder J-M (1995) Detection of chemokine RANTES in stimulated human dermal fibroblasts. *J Invest Dermatol* 105: 585–591

29 Noso N, Sticherling M, Bartels J, Mallet AI, Christophers E, Schröder J-M (1996) Identification of an NH$_2$-terminally truncated form of the chemokine RANTES and GM-CSF as major eosinophil attractants released by cytokine-stimulated dermal fibroblasts. *J Immunol* 156: 1946–1953

30 Marfaing-Koka A, Devergne O, Gorgone G, Portier A, Schall TJ, Galanaud P, Emilie D (1995) Regulation of the production of the RANTES chemokine by endothelial cells. *J Immunol* 154: 1870–1878

31 Kapp A, Zeck Kapp G, Czech W, Schopf E (1994) The chemokine RANTES is more than a chemoattractant: characterization of its effect on human eosinophil oxidative

metabolism and morphology in comparison with IL-5 and GM-CSF. *J Invest Dermatol* 102: 906–914

32 Meurer R, Van Riper G, Feeney W, Cunningham P, Hora D Jr, Springer MS, McIntyre DR, Rosen H (1993) Formation of eosinophilic and monocytic intradermal inflammatory sites in the dog by injection of human RANTES but not human monocyte chemoattractant protein 1, human macrophage inflammatory protein 1 alpha, or human interleukin 8. *J Exp Med* 178: 1913–1921

33 Rohde D, Stampor V, Langner A, Christophers E (1994) Cutaneous inflammation mediated by intradermal injection of RANTES and FMLP. Ultrastructural and immunohistochemical features. *J Invest Dermatol* 103: 425

34 Noso N, Proost P, Van Damme J, Schröder J-M (1994) Human monocyte chemotactic proteins-2 and 3 (MCP-2 and MCP-3) attract human eosinophils and desensitize the chemotactic responses towards RANTES. *Biochem Biophys Res Commun* 200: 1470–1476

35 Weber M, Uguccioni M, Ochensberger B, Baggiolini M, Clark-Lewis I, Dahinden CA (1995) Monocyte chemotactic protein MCP-2 activates human basophil and eosinophil leukocytes similar to MCP-3. *J Immunol* 154: 4166–4172

36 Chang HC, Hsu F, Freeman GJ, Griffin JD, Reinherz EL (1989) Cloning and expression of a γ-interferon-inducible gene in monocytes: A new member of a cytokine gene family. *Int Immunol* 1: 388–397

37 Van Damme J, Proost P, Put W, Arens S, Lenaerts JP, Conings R, Opdenakker G, Heremans H, Billiau A (1994) Induction of monocyte chemotactic proteins MCP-1 and MCP-2 in human fibroblasts and leukocytes by cytokines and cytokine inducers. Chemical synthesis of MCP-2 and development of a specific RIA. *J Immunol* 152: 5495–5502

38 Kulmburg PA, Huber NE, Scheer BJ, Wrann M, Baumruker T (1992) Immunoglobuline E plus antigen challenge induces a novel intercrine/chemokine in mouse mast cells. *J Exp Med* 176: 1773–1778

39 Dahinden CA, Geiser T, Brunner T, von Tscharner V, Caput D, Ferrara P, Minty A, Baggiolini M (1994) Monocyte chemotactic protein 3 is a most effective basophil- and eosinophil-activating chemokine. *J Exp Med* 179: 751–756

38 Van Damme J, Proost P, Lenaerts JP, Opdenakker G (1992) Structural and functional identification of two human, tumor-derived monocyte chemotactic proteins (MCP-2 and MCP-3) belonging to the chemokine family. *J Exp Med* 176: 59–65

39 Uguccioni M, Loetscher P, Forssmann U, Dewald B, Li HD, Lima SH, Li YL, Kreider B, Garotta G, Thelen M, Baggiolini M (1996) Monocyte chemotactic protein 4 (MCP-4), a novel structural and functional analogue of MCP-3 and eotaxin. *J Exp Med* 183: 2379–2384

40 Jose PJ, Griffiths-Johnson DA, Collins PD, Walsh DT, Moqbel R, Totty NF, Truong O, Hsuan JJ, Williams TJ (1994) Eotaxin: a potent eosinophil chemoattractant cytokine detected in a guinea pig model of allergic airways inflammation. *J Exp Med* 179: 881–887

41 Rothenberg ME, Luster AD, Leder P (1995) Murine eotaxin: an eosinophil chemoat-tractant inducible in endothelial cells and in interleukin 4-induced tumor suppression. *Proc Natl Acad Sci USA* 92: 8960–8964

42 Ponath PD, Qin S, Ringler DJ, Clark-Lewis I, Wang J, Kassam N, Smith H, Shi X, Gon-zalo JA, Newman W, Gutierrez-Ramos JC, Mackay CR (1996) Cloning of the human eosinophil chemoattractant, Eotaxin. *J Clin Invest* 97: 604–612

43 Garcia-Zepeda EA, Rothenberg ME, Ownbey RT, Celestin J, Leder P, Luster AD (1996) Human eotaxin is a specific chemoattractant for eosinophil cells and provides a new mechanism to explain tissue eosinophilia. *Nature Medicine* 2: 449-456

44 Kitaura M, Nakajima T, Imai T, Harada S, Combadiere C, Tiffany HL, Murphy PM, Yoshie O (1996) Molecular cloning of human eotaxin, an eosinophil-selective CC chemokine, and identification of a specific eosinophil eotaxin receptor, CC chemokine receptor 3. *J Biol Chem* 271: 7725–7730

45 Lilly CM, Nakamura H, Kesselman H, Nagler-Anderson C, Asano K, GarciaZepeda EA, Rothenberg ME, Drazen JM, Luster AD (1997) Expression of eotaxin by human lung epithelial cells – Induction by cytokines and inhibition by glucocorticoids. *J Clin Invest* 99: 1767–1773

46 Bartels J, Schlüter C, Richter E, Noso N, Kulke R, Christophers E, Schröder J-M (1996) Human dermal fibroblasts express eotaxin: molecular cloning, mRNA expression, and identification of eotaxin sequence variants. *Biochem Biophys Res Commun* 225: 1045–1051

47 Forssmann U, Uguccioni M, Loetscher P, Dahinden CA, Langen H, Thelen M, Baggi-olini M (1997) Eotaxin-2, a novel CC chemokine that is selective for the chemokine receptor CCR3, and acts like eotaxin on human eosinophil and basophil leukocytes. *J Exp Med* 185: 2171–2176

48 Elsner J, Höchstetter R, Kimmig D, Kapp A (1996) Human eotaxin represents a potent activator of the respiratory burst of human eosinophils. *Eur J Immunol* 26: 1919–1925

49 Schweizer RC, Welmers BAC, Raaijmakers JAM, Zanen P, Lammers JW, Koenderman L (1994) Rantes- and interleukin-8-induced responses in normal human eosinophils: effects of priming with interleukin-5. *Blood* 83: 3697–3704

50 Baggiolini M, Dewald B, Moser B (1997) Human chemokines: An update. *Annu Rev Immunol* 15: 675–705

51 Baggiolini M, Dahinden CA (1994) CC chemokines in allergic inflammation. *Immuno-logy Today* 15: 127–133

52 Heath H, Qin SX, Rao P, Wu LJ, LaRosa G, Kassam N, Ponath PD, Makay CR (1997) Chemokine receptor usage by human eosinophils – The importance of CCR3 de-monstrated using an antagonistic monoclonal antibody. *J Clin Invest* 99: 178–184

53 Schröder J-M, Noso N, Sticherling M, Christophers E (1996) Role of eosinophil-chemotactic C-C chemokines in cutaneous inflammation. *J Leuko Biol* 59: 1–5

54 Schröder J-M, Mrowietz U, Morita E, Christophers E (1987) Purification and partial

biochemical characterization of a human monocyte-derived, neutrophil activating pepti-de that lacks interleukin 1 activity. *J Immunol* 139: 3474–3483

55 Sehmi R, Cromwell O, Wardlaw AJ, Moqbel R, Kay AB (1993) Interleukin-8 is a chemo-attractant for eosinophils purified from subjects with a blood eosinophilia but not from normal healthy subjects. *Clin Exp Allergy* 23: 1027–1036

56 Moqbel R, Levi-Schaffer F, Kay AB (1994) Cytokine generation by eosinophils. *J Allergy Clin Immunol* 94: Suppl. 1183–1188

57 Braun RK, Franchini M, Erard F, Rihs S, De Vries IJM, Blaser K, Hansel TT, Walker C (1993) Human peripheral blood eosinophils produce and release interleukin-8 on stim-ulation with calcium ionophore. *Eur J Immunol* 23: 956–960

58 Miyamasu M, Hirai K, Takahashi Y, Iida M, Yamaguchi M, Koshino T, Takaishi T, Morita Y, Ohta K, Kasahara T, Ito K (1995) Chemotactic agonists induce cytokine gen-eration in eosinophils. *J Immunol* 154: 1339–1349

59 Costa JJ, Matossian K, Resnick MB, Beil WJ, Wong DTW, Gordon JR, Dvorak AM, Weller PF, Galli SJ (1993) Human eosinophils can express the cytokines tumor necrosis factor-α and macrophage inflammatory protein-1α. *J Clin Invest* 91: 2673–2684

60 Izumi S, Hirai K, Miyamasu M, Takahashi Y, Misaki Y, Takaishi T, Morita Y, Mat-sushima K, Ida N, Nakamura H, Kasahara T, Ito K (1997) Expression and regulation of monocyte chemoattractant protein-1 by human eosinophils. *Eur J Immunol* 27: 816–824

61 Ying S, Taborda-Barata L, Meng Q, Humbert M, Kay AB (1995) The kinetics of aller-gen-induced transcription of messenger RNA for monocyte chemotactic protein-3 and RANTES in the skin of human atopic subjects: relationship to eosinophil, T cell, and macrophage recruitment. *J Exp Med* 181: 2153–2159

62 Schall TJ, Bacon K, Toy KJ, Goeddel DV (1990) Selective attraction on monocytes and T lymphocytes of the memory phenotype by cytokine RANTES. *Nature* 347: 669–671

63 Sur S, Kita H, Gleich GJ, Chenier TC, Hunt LW (1996) Eosinophil recruitment is asso-ciated with IL-5, but not with RANTES, twenty-four hours after allergen challenge. *J Allergy Clin Immunol* 97: 1272–1278

64 Schrum S, Probst P, Fleischer B, Zipfel PF (1996) Synthesis of the CC-chemokines MIP-1α, MIP-1β and RANTES is associated with a Type I immune response. *J Immunol* 157: 3598–3604

65 Rankin JA, Picarella DE, Geba GP, Temann UA, Prasad B, DiCosmo B, Tarallo A, Stripp B, Whitsett J, Flavell RA (1996) Phenotypic and physiologic characterization of trans-genic mice expressing interleukin 4 in the lung: Lymphocytic and eosinophilic inflamma-tion without airway hyperreactivity. *Proc Natl Acad Sci USA* 93: 7821–7824

66 Pearlman E, Lass JH, Bardenstein DS, Diaconu E, Hazlett FE, Albright J, Higgins AW, Kazura JW (1996) Onchocerca volvulus-mediated keratitis: cytokine production by IL-4-deficient mice. *Exp Parasitol* 84: 274–281

67 Brusselle G, Kips J, Joos G, Bluethmann H, Pauwels R (1995) Allergen-induced airway inflammation and bronchial responsiveness in wild type and interleukin-4-deficient mice. *Am J Respir Cell Mol Biol* 12: 254–261

68 Mochizuki M, Bartels J, Mallet AI, Christophers E, Schröder J-M (1998) IL-4 induces eotaxin: a possible mechanism of selective eosinophil recruitment in helminth infection and atopy. *J Immunol* 160: 60–68

69 Locksley RM (1994) Th2 cells: Help for helminths. *J Exp Med* 179: 1405–1407

70 Bradding P, Feather IH, Howarth PH, Mueller R, Roberts JA, Britten K, Bews JPA, Hunt TC, Okayama Y, Heusser CH, Bullock GR, Church MK, Holgate ST (1992) Interleukin 4 is localized to and released by human mast cells. *J Exp Med* 176: 1381–1386

71 Schall TJ, Bacon KB (1994) Chemokines, leukocyte trafficking, and inflammation. *Curr Opin Immunol* 6: 865–873

72 Gonzalo JA, Lloyd CM, Kremer L, Finger E, Martinez C, Siegelman MH, Cybulsky M, Gutierrez-Ramos JC (1996) Eosinophil recruitment to the lung in a murine model of allergic inflammation – The role of T cells, chemokines, and adhesion receptors. *J Clin Invest* 98: 2332–2345

CXC-Chemokines – autocrine growth factors for melanoma and epidermoid carcinoma cells

Beatrix Metzner, Frank Peters, Clemens Hofmann, Ulrich Zimpfer and Johannes Norgauer

Department of Experimental Dermatology, University of Freiburg, Hauptstr. 7,
D-79104 Freiburg, Germany

Cells of the epidermis

The epidermis is a multi-layered epithelium forming the interface between the body and its environment. Keratinocytes are the predominant cell population of this layer. They provide the barrier between the body and the enviroment. They originate from the superficial ectoderm of the implanted embryo [1, 2]. The other major cells of the epidermis are melanocytes. They are secretory neural crest-derived cells uniquely located within the basal layer of the epidermis and in the matrix of hair follicles. During fetal development melanocytes migrate into the skin and inhabit the epidermis as a fixed cell population [3]. The fully differentiated human melanocyte synthesizes melanin and transfers pigment-containing organelles to surrounding keratinocytes [4]. Melanization is responsible for skin tanning and provide protection against ultraviolet irradiation [5].

Growth control mechanisms of keratinocytes and melanocytes

The growth of keratinocytes and melanocytes in the epidermis is controlled by a complex interaction of different molecules [6, 7]. The signals include soluble factors and cell-cell contacts [8]. Proliferation of keratinocytes in the epidermis is presumably regulated by paracrine secretion of transforming growth factor α and by soluble factors released from fibroblasts such as keratinocyte growth factor and interleukin-6 [9]. Secreted peptides by keratinocytes such as basic fibroblast growth factor, endothelin-1, α-melanocyte-stimulating hormone and granulocyte-macrophage colony-stimulating factor are well characterized growth factors for melanocytes [10, 11]. The mechanisms and the receptors involved in the control of proliferation of keratinocytes and melanocytes by cell-cell contact are largely unknown. However, a regulatory role of keratinocytes for melanocytic cells appears to work at several levels [10]. Keratinocytes induce to adapt melanocytes a dendritic morphology.

In tissue culture experiments a constant keratinocyte/melanocyte ratio is maintained during the exponential growth phase [12].

Transformation and autocrine growth loops

Tranformed and malignant cells evade growth control of the physiological microenviroment by establishing autocrine stimulatory loops. Overexpression and synthesis of the epidermal growth factor receptor and its ligand transforming growth factor α plays a role in the serum-independent growth of transformed keratinocytes derived from squamous cell carcinoma [13, 14]. A similar overexpression mechanism is known in melanoma cells involving basic fibroblast growth factor and its receptor *flg*-1 [15, 16]. There is also evidence that overexpression of the CXC-chemokines interleukin-8 (IL-8) and growth related oncogene α (GROα) as well as their receptors contribute to the transformed phenotype of melanoma cells [17–23].

Relation between inflammation and squamous cell carcinoma

Squamous cell carcinoma occur with increased frequency at sites of chronic inflammation such as long-lasting crural ulcers, persistent fistulas and lesions of lupus vulgaris as well as sun-exposed regions [24]. It is tempting to speculate that mediators of the inflammatory response and ultraviolet radiation-induced genes might function as tumor promoters for keratinocytes.

Attractive candidates participating in the tumorgenesis of squamous cell carcinoma are CXC-chemokines. They are usually highly expressed at sites of inflammation [25, 26]. Expression and synthesis of the CXC-chemokines are induced by environmental factors such as ultraviolet radiation [27]. Increased CXC-chemokine immunoreactivity is also detected in biopsy specimens of squamous cell carcinoma [28]. Tissue culture experiments performed in multiple groups reveal high constitutive production of CXC-chemokines in epidermoid carcinoma cells in contrast to their normal counterparts [25]. Recent studies suggest that IL-8 and GROα might not only influence leukocytes but also stimulate different functions of keratinocytes such as chemotaxis and HLA-DR expression [29, 30]. It appears that overexpressed CXC-chemokines in epidermoid carcinoma cell might function as growth factors [18, 28].

However, a series of clinical observations argue against such a simple model of pathogenesis of the squamous cell carcinoma. Formation of squamous cell carcinoma is not enhanced in lesions of psoriasis vulgaris and pustulosis palmoplantaris, where overexpression of CXC-chemokines is a constant finding [31]. In tissue culture experiments only a weak growth proliferative activity of CXC-chemokines on normal keratinocytes is detected [32].

CXC-chemokine receptors

CXC-chemokines signal by binding to two hepta-helical rhodopsin-like G-Protein-coupled receptors, named CXC-receptor 1 (CXCR1) and CXC-receptor 2 (CXCR2) [33–36]. Interleukin-8 binds to both receptors with high affinity, whereas GROα has high affinity for CXCR2 and low affinity for CXCR1. Cell activation requires high affinity ligand binding. No activity at physiologically relevant concentrations was found with low affinity binding of GROα to CXCR1 [37–39].

To identify the function of CXC-chemokines in normal keratinocytes and in their malignant counterparts we performed binding experiments. These experiments revealed no statistically significant binding of [^{125}I]IL-8 or [^{125}I]GROα to normal keratinocytes. However, a single class of high affinity binding sites for GROα and IL-8 was detected in epidermoid carcinoma cells (Fig. 1). Since GROα binds with high affinity to CXCR2 and with low affinity to CXCR1 the presence of only CXCR2 on these cells was assumed. This conclusion could be further corroborated by flow cytometric analysis using iso-type specific antibodies with ligand binding properties. Again no significant expression of CXCR1 and CXCR2 was found on the cell surface of normal keratinocytes (Tab.1). However, the epidermoid carcinoma cells KB and A431 expressed high levels of CXCR2 at the cell surface. No expression of CXCR1 in epidermoid carcinoma cells was seen.

Table 1 - Expression of the CXCR2 in different epidermoid carcinoma cell lines and keratinocytes

Cell line	Control[a]	anti-CXCR2[a]	anti-CXCR1[a]
Keratinocytes	69 ± 4	112 ± 8	79 ± 5
KB	73 ± 3	1107 ± 23	98 ± 7
A431	88 ± 5	2373 ± 26	104 ± 10

[a] *Mean channel number of stained F(ab')$_2$-fragments from control, anti-CXCR2 antiserum or anti-CXCR1 antiserum. KB and A431 are epidermoid carcinoma cells. Data are means ± SEM (n=3)*

Overexpression of CXCR2 and autocrine growth loops in epidermoid carcinoma cells

To study the growth-stimulating properties of CXC-chemokines, [^{3}H]thymidine incorporation into normal keratinocytes or epidermoid carcinoma cells was quantified. Thereby we found that CXC-chemokines had no significant influence on the

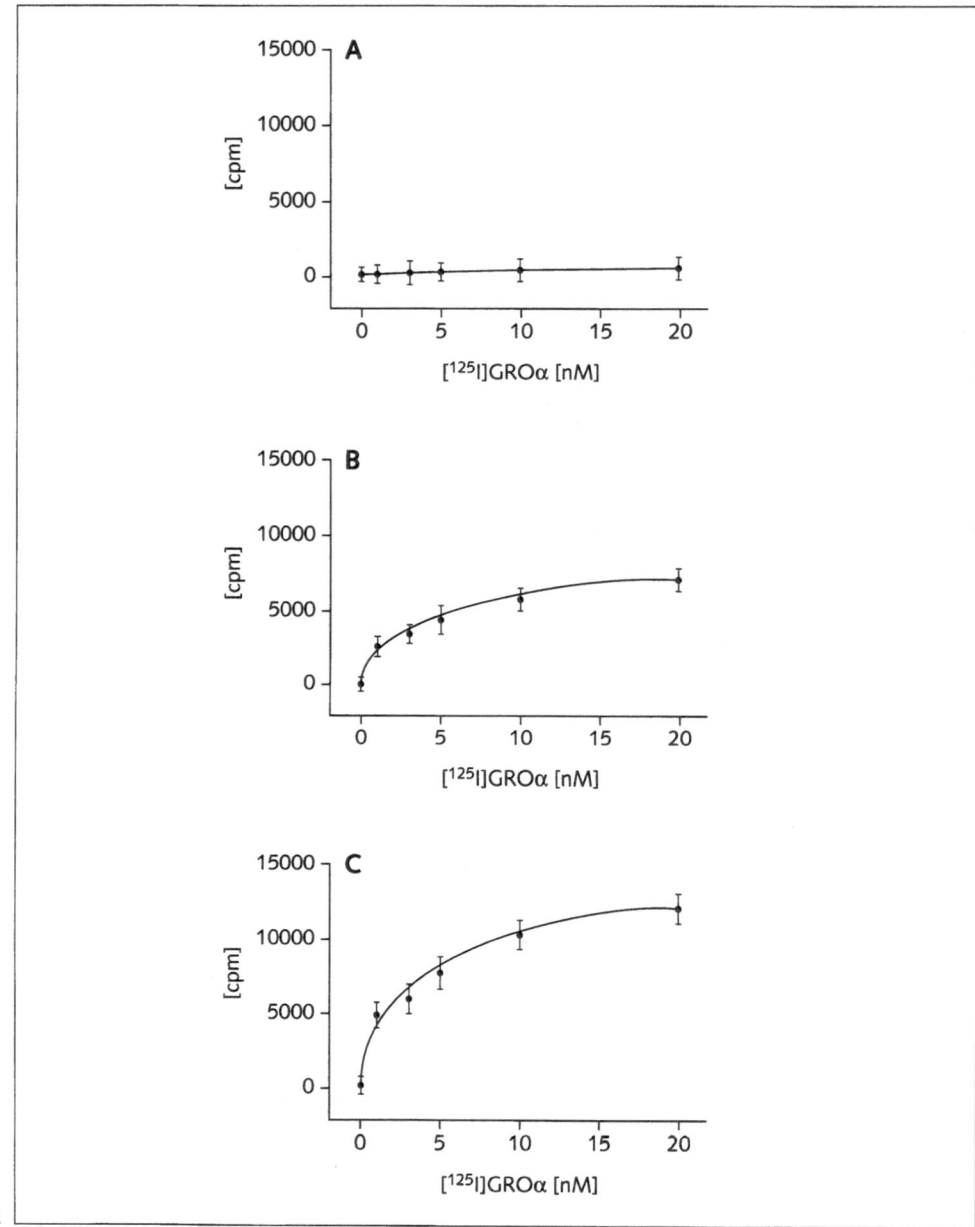

1A

Figure 1

Binding of [^{125}I]GROα (Fig. 1A) and [^{125}I]IL-8 (Fig. 1B) in normal keratinocytes (A) and epidermoid carcinoma cell KB (B) and A431. Cells were incubated with the indicated concentrations of [^{125}I]GROα and [^{125}I]IL-8 in the presence or absence of 1000-fold excess of unlabeled ligands. Specific binding of both ligands to the cells were calculated. Data are means ± SEM (n=3)

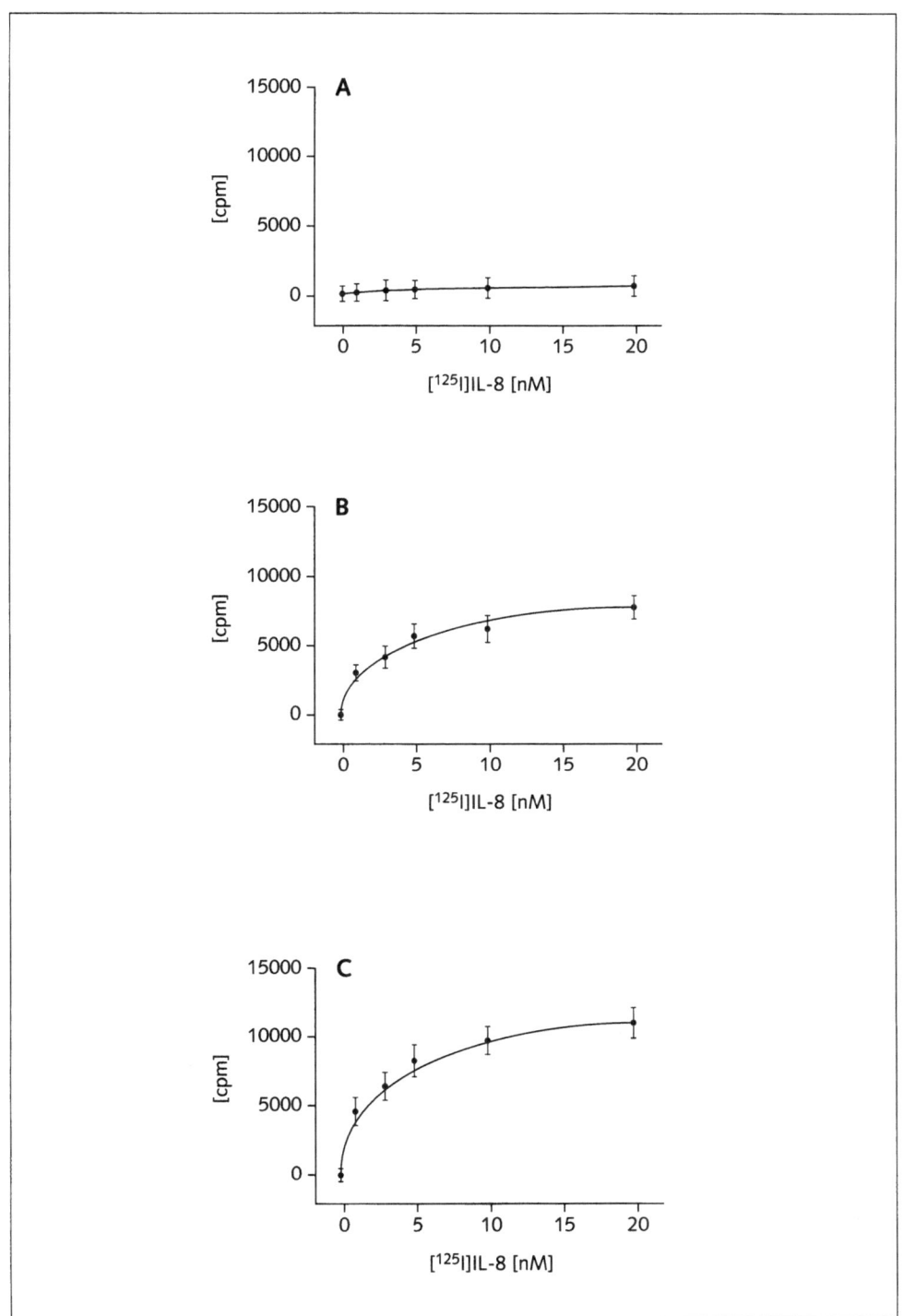

1B

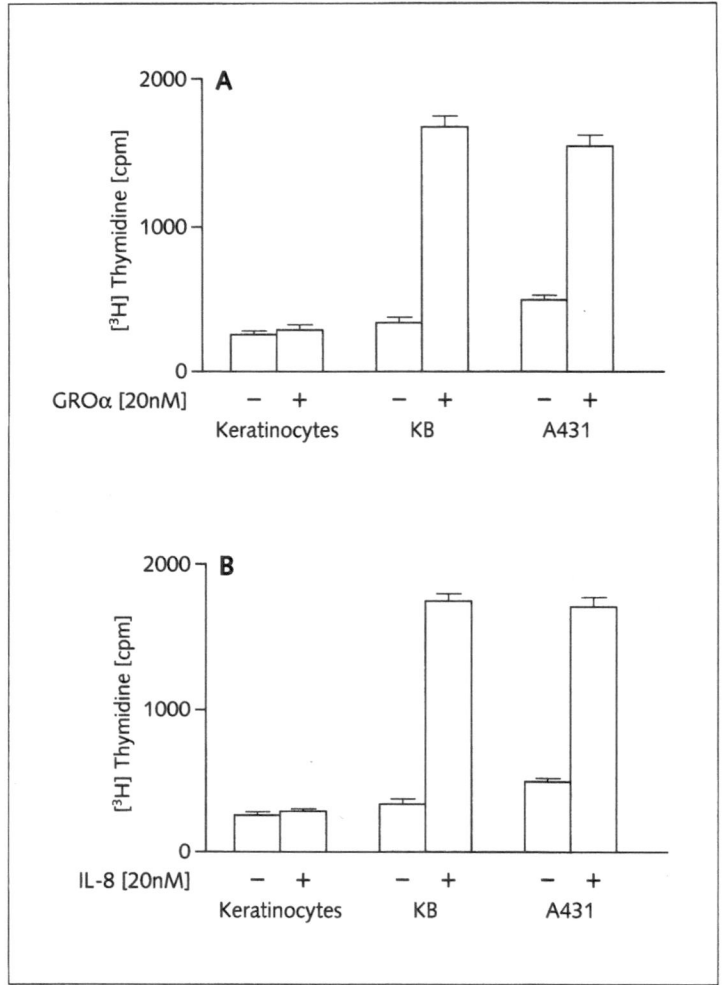

Figure 2
Influence of GROα (Fig. 2A) and IL-8 (Fig. 2B) on proliferation of normal keratinocytes and epidermoid carcinoma cells (KB, A431). The cells (50 000 cells/well) were stimulated with 20 nM GROα or 20 nM IL-8. Incorporation of [³H]thymidine was determined. Data are means ± SEM (n=4).

proliferation of normal keratinocytes, whereas a concentration-dependent stimulation was found in epidermoid carcinoma cells (Fig. 2). These comparisons indicate that overexpression of CXCR2 enabled CXC-chemokines to function as growth factors for epidermoid carcinoma cells.

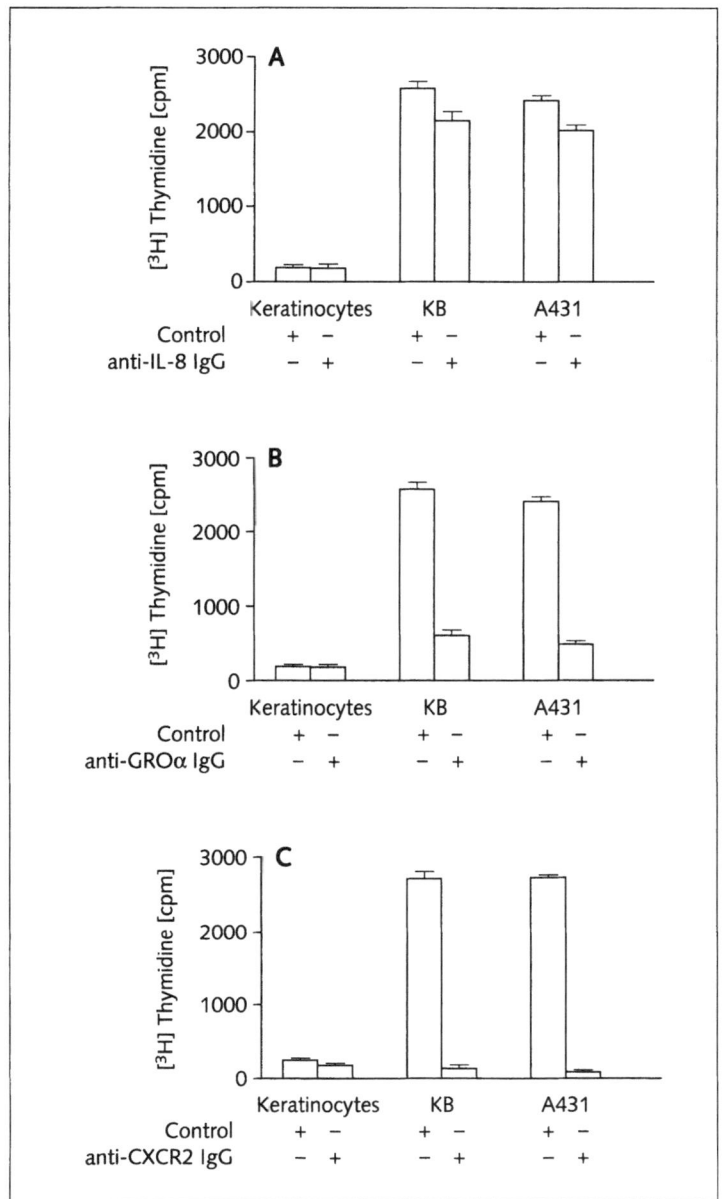

Figure 3
Effect of monoclonal anti-human IL-8 IgG (A) and monoclonal anti-human GROα IgG (B) and anti-CXCR2 IgG (C) on growth of normal keratinocytes and epidermoid carcinoma cells. Serum-starved cells (50 000 cells/well) were incubated with 1 mg/ml anti-human IL-8 IgG, 1 mg/ml anti-GROα IgG and 2 mg/ml anti-CXCR2 IgG or irrelevant isotype-specific control antibodies for 24 h. Incorporation of [³H]thymidine was analyzed. Data are means ± SEM (n=4).

Since transformed epidermoid carcinoma cells constitutively synthesize CXC-chemokines the influence of blocking antibodies against CXC-chemokines and CXCR2 was studied. Using these tools we could inhibit constitutive proliferation of epidermoid carcinoma cells (Fig. 3). These data strongly indicate that CXC-chemokines and CXCR2 are essential components of an autocrine growth loop in epidermoid carcinoma cells.

CXC-chemokines and receptors – therapeutic targets in skin cancer?

CXC-chemokines are well established molecules provoking inflammation. The data presented suggest that they have a broader physiological relevance than previously realised. They appear to play an essential role in the growth of melanoma cells and transformed keratinocytes, while the benign counterparts neither produced nor responded to CXC-chemokines. If the overexpression of CXC-chemokines and their receptor were a unique property of the malignant cells this could be a candidate for therapeutic intervention.

Usually malignant cells do not express entirely new properties, but differ from the original cells quantitatively. It is conceivable that cell culture techniques deprive the benign cells of an essential cofactor, which the malignant cells do not depend on. To analyse this the cell culture would need to imitate more closely the situation *in vivo* with cell contacts and other cytokines present.

References

1   Holbrook KA (1994) Ultrastructure of the epidermis. In: I Leigh, B Lane, F Watt (eds): *The keratinocyte handbook*. Cambridge University Press, Cambridge, 3–39

2   Mitra R, Nickoloff B (1994) Cultivation of human epidermal keratinocytes in serum-free growth medium. In: I Leigh, F Watt (eds): *Keratinocyte methods*. Cambridge University Press, Cambridge, 17–19

3   Hirobe T (1995) Structure and function of melanocytes: microscopic morphology and cell biology of mouse melanocytes in the epidermis and hair follicle. *Histo Histophath* 10: 223–237

4   Morelli JG, Norris DA (1993) Influence of inflammatory mediators and cytokines on human melanocyte function. *J Invest Dermatol* 100: 191S–195S

5   De Luca M, Bondanza S, Di Marco E, Marchisio PC, D'Anna F, Franzi AT, Cancedda R (1994) Keratinocyte-melanocyte interactions in in vitro reconstituted normal human epidermis. In: I Leigh, B Lane, F Watt (eds): *The keratinocyte handbook*. Cambridge University Press, Cambridge, 95–108

6   Stoff TJ, Boorsma DM, Nickoloff BJ (1994) Keratinocytes and immunological

cytokines. In: I Leigh, B Lane, F Watt (eds): *The keratinocyte handbook*. Cambridge University Press, Cambridge, 365–399

7   MacKenzie IC (1994) Epithelial-mesenchymal interactions in the development and maintenance of epithelial tissue. In: I Leigh, B Lane, F Watt (eds): *The keratinocyte handbook*. Cambridge University Press, Cambridge, 243–258

8   Herlyn M, Shih IM (1994) Interactions of melanocytes and melanoma cells with the microenvironment. *Pigment Cell Res* 7: 81–88

9   Fusenig NE (1994) Epithelial-mesenchymal interactions regulate keratinocyte growth and differentiation *in vitro*. In: I Leigh, B Lane, F Watt (eds): *The keratinocyte handbook*. Cambridge University Press, Cambridge, 71–94

10 Gordon PR, Mansur CP, Gilchrest BA (1989) Regulation of human melanocyte growth, dendricity, and melanization by keratinocyte derived factors. *J Invest Dermatol* 9: 565–572

11 Imokawa G, Yada Y, Kimura M, Morisaki N (1996) Granulocyte/macrophage colony-stimulating factor is an intrinsic keratinocyte-derived growth factor for human melanocytes in UVA-induced melanosis. *Biochem J* 313: 625–631

12 Luger TA, Schwarz T (1990) Evidence for an epidermal cytokine network. *J Invest Dermatol* 96: 100S–104S

13 Moroni MC, Willingham MC, Beguinot L (1992) EGF-R antisense RNA blocks expression of the epidermal growth factor receptor and suppresses the transforming phenotype of a human carcinoma cell line. *J Biol Chem* 267: 2714–2722

14 Nicolini G, Miloso M, Moroni MC, Beguinot L, Scotto L (1996) Post-transcriptional control regulates transforming growth factor α in the human carcinoma KB cell line. *J Biol Chem* 271: 30290–30296

15 Becker D, Meier CB, Herlyn M (1989) Proliferation of human malignant melanomas is inhibited by antisense oligodeoxynucleotides targeted against basic fibroblast growth factor. *EMBO J* 8: 3685–3691

16 Becker D, Lee PL, Rodeck U, Herlyn M (1992) Inhibition of the fibroblast growth factor receptor-1 (FGFR-1) gene in human melanocytes and malignant melanomas leads to inhibition of proliferation and signs indicative of differentiation. *Oncogene* 7: 2303–2313

17 Lawson DH, Thomas HG, Roy RGB, Gordon DS, Chawla RK, Nixon DW, Richmond A (1987) Preparation of a monoclonal antibody to a melanoma growth stimulatory activity released into serum-free culture medium by Hs294T malignant melanoma cells. *J Cell Biochem* 34: 169–185

18 Richmond A, Balentien E, Thomas HG, Flaggs G, Barton DE, Spiess J, Bordoni R, Francke U, Derynck R (1988) Molecular characterization and chromosal mapping of melanoma growth stimulatory activity, a growth factor structurally related to β-thromboglobulin. *EMBO J* 7: 2025–2033

19 Bordoni R, Fine R, Murray D, Richmond A (1990) Characterization of the role of melanoma growth stimulatory activity (MGSA) in the growth of normal melanocytes, nevocytes, and malignant melanocytes. *J Cell Biochem* 44: 207–219

20 Schadendorf D, Möller A, Algermissen B, Worm M, Sticherling M, Czarnetzki BM (1993) IL-8 produced by human malignant melanoma cells in vitro is an essential autocrine growth factor. *J Immunol* 151: 2667–2675

21 Krasagakis K, Garbe C, Orfanos CE (1993) Cytokines in human melanoma cells: synthesis, autocrine stimulation and regulatory functions – an overview. *Melanoma Res 3*: 425–433

22 Krasagakis K, Garbe C, Zouboulis CC, Orfanos CE (1995) Growth control of melanoma cells and melanocytes by cytokines. *Rec Res in Canc Res* 139: 169–182

23 Norgauer J, Metzner B, Schraufstätter I (1996) Expression and growth-promoting function of the IL-8 receptor β in human melanoma cells. *J Immunol* 156: 1132–1137

24 Braun-Falco O, Plewig G, Wolff HH, Winkelmann RK (1991) *Dermatology.* Springer-Verlag, Berlin, 1019–1035

25 Baggiolini M, Loetscher P, Moser B (1995) Interleukin-8 and the chemokine family. *Int J of Immunopharm* 17: 103–108

26 Proost P, Wuyts A, van Damme J (1996) The role of chemokines in inflammation. *Int J Clin Lab Res* 26: 211–223

27 Venner TJ, Sauder DN, Feliciani C, Mckenzie RC (1995) Interleukin-8 and melanoma growth-stimulating activity (GRO) are induced by ultraviolet B radiation in human keratinocyte cell lines. *Exp Dermat* 4, 138–145

28 Tettelbach W, Nannely L, Ellis E, King L, Richmond A (1993) Localization of MGSA/GROα protein in cutaneous lesions. *J Cut Pathol* 20: 259–266

29 Michel G, Kenemy L, Peter RO, Beetz A, Ried C, Arenberger P, Ruzicka T (1992) Interleukin-8 receptor mediated chemotaxis of normal human epidermal cells. *FEBS Lett* 305: 241–243

30 Kemeny L, Kenderessy AS, Ocsovszky I, Michel G, Ruzicka T, Dobozy A (1995) Interleukin-8 induces HLA-DR expession on cultured human keratinocytes via specific receptors. *Int Arch Allergy Immunol* 106: 351–356

31 Schröder J-M (1992) Chemotactic cytokines in the epidermis. *Exp Dermatol* 1: 12–19

32 Tuschil A, Lam C, Haslberger A, Lindley I (1992) Interleukin-8 stimulates calcium transients and promotes epidermal cell proliferation. *J Invest Dermatol* 99: 294–298

33 Murphy PM, Tiffany HL (1991) Cloning of complementary DNA encoding a functional interleukin-8 receptor. *Science* 253: 1280–1282

34 Holmes WE, Lee J, Kuang WJ, Rice GC, Wood WI (1991) Structure and expression of a human interleukin-8 receptor. *Science* 253: 1278–1280

35 Ahuja SK, Gao J-L, Murphy PM (1994) Chemokine receptors and molecular mimicry. *Immunol Today* 15: 281-287

36 Ahuja SK, Lee JC, Murphy PM (1996) CXC chemokines bind to unique sets of selectivity determinants that can function independently and are broadly distributed on multiple domains of human interleukin-8 receptor B Determinants of high affinity binding and receptor activation are distinct. *J Biol Chem* 271: 225–232

37 LaRosa GJ, Thomas KM, Kaufmann ME, Mark R, White M, Taylor L, Gray G, Witt D,

Navarro J (1992) Amino terminus of the interleukin-8 receptor is a major determinant of receptor subtype specifity. *J Biol Chem* 267: 25002–25006

38   Schraufstätter IU, Barritt DS, Ma Z, Oades ZG, Cochrane CG (1993) Multiple sites on IL-8 responsible for binding to α and β IL-8 receptors. *J Immunol* 151: 6418–6428

39   Loetscher P, Seitz M, Clark-Lewis I, Baggiolini M, Moser B (1994) Both interleukin-8 receptors independently mediate chemotaxis. *FEBS Lett* 341: 187–192

Expression of chemokines in dermatoses

Reinhard Gillitzer, Eva Engelhardt and Matthias Goebeler

Department of Dermatology, University of Würzburg Medical School, D-97080 Würzburg, Germany

Introduction

Most skin disorders (dermatoses), with the rare exception of some congenital or metabolic diseases and tumors with low or absent antigenicity, are characterised by a concomitant inflammatory reaction. The composition of inflammatory cell infiltrates as well as their tissue distribution may reflect the pathogenesis of a particular disease and are important hallmarks for histological diagnosis.

For a long time scientists wondered about the signals that could specifically draw a given cell into a given tissue. With the identification of interleukin 8 (IL-8) [1–5] and monocyte chemoattractant protein-1 (MCP-1) [6, 7] proteins were described that were able to specifically deliver migratory signals to distinct cell types, e.g. neutrophils and monocytes. While our understanding of the functions of the prototype chemokines IL-8 and MCP-1 has been significantly extended in recent years through detailed *in vitro* and *in vivo* studies, the role of most chemokines in physiological and pathological processes remains to be elucidated.

Invasion of leukocytes always follows the route from the lumen of a dermal vessel into the dermal milieu and possibly further on to the epidermal compartment. Thus, migration of inflammatory cells across several compartment borders is unique and presents an ideal model for evaluation of chemotactic cytokine functions *in vivo*. Moreover, the unidirectional migration pattern of cells along an increasing chemoattractant gradient justifies the concept that the dermal and/or epidermal expression of chemotactic components and chemokines in particular accounts for the distribution and composition of inflammatory cell infiltrates in skin disorders. This chapter illuminates the role of chemokines in various skin disorders with particular emphasis on inflammatory skin diseases.

Chemokines and Skin, edited by E. Kownatzki and J. Norgauer
© 1998 Birkhäuser Verlag Basel/Switzerland

Chemokine expression in inflammatory skin disorders

The cellular composition and tissue distribution of inflammatory cell infiltrates, assist dermatopathologists in specifically diagnosing inflammatory skin diseases. According to the chemoattractant function of chemokines, it is tempting to speculate that the cellular infiltration pattern in inflammatory skin disorders mirrors the expression pattern of chemokines. This holds true for psoriasis, where the first chemokine, IL-8, has been discovered [1] and the *in vivo* expression of chemokines been studied in detail [8–10, 37]. Regarding other inflammatory reactions (e.g. lichen planus, erythema multiforme, graft versus host reactions, contact dermatitis, atopic eczema, lupus erythematosus), our knowledge about lesional chemokine production is rather restricted.

Chemokine expression in psoriasis

The best studied inflammatory disease in humans is probably psoriasis. It is characterised by a regio-specific infiltration of leukocytes. Whereas neutrophils multifocally and rapidly cross the dermal compartment and migrate a long distance to the uppermost layer of the acanthotic epidermis forming microabscesses and pustules, macrophages reside in the dermis with a subpopulation lining up below the basement membrane of the rete ridges. These macrophages are termed "lining cells" and are in close contact with the hyperproliferative basal keratinocytes. T cells are encountered in the dermis and epidermis, with a predominance of CD8 positive cells in the epidermis.

The accumulation of neutrophils in the uppermost part of the epidermis has been explained by a staggered gradient of IL-8 and GRO [12, 13], whereas mRNA expression of another neutrophil-attractant CXC chemokine, ENA-78 [11], was found to be absent [10]. Among the three different GRO subtypes GROα appears to be selectively overexpressed [14]. A possible scenario for leukocyte recruitment in psoriasis is depicted in Figure 1. Initially, neutrophils interact with various luminal adhesion-promoting glycoproteins (i.e. intercellular adhesion molecule-1, vascular cell adhesion molecule-1, E-selectin) resulting in rolling along the vessel walls and adhesion to the dermal endothelium [15]. Thereafter, neutrophils migrate through the endothelial wall. They appear to be directed by GROα which is synthesised by dermal endothelial as well as by dermal perivascular mononuclear cells [16].

Although previous publications favor IL-8 as the locomotor attractant for neutrophils during diapedesis [17], IL-8 message has never been detected in dermal endothelial cells *in vivo* (our own observation). In the dermis, neutrophils pick up a gradient of both IL-8 and GROα produced by upper level keratinocytes and migrate to the stratum corneum (see Fig. 1). The regulation of the chemokine receptors

CXCR1 and CXCR2 on neutrophils *in vivo* is not known, but both chemokines have an overlapping but also distinctive receptor specificity (see I.U. Schraufstätter et al., this volume). Possibly, initial receptor desensitisation of the IL-8 receptor B (CXCR2) through GROα may be overcome through IL-8 and activation of the IL-8 receptorA (CXCR1) [18–21]. This observation together with the differential expression of IL-8 and GROα might explain the capability of neutrophils to migrate a long distance through several compartments and their rapid recruitment to sites of inflammatory disturbances.

In psoriasis, neutrophils are directed multifocally to the outermost part of the epidermis which is well in accordance with the multifocal and periodical expression of IL-8 and GROα. Besides the function of IL-8 as a potent neutrophil chemoattractant, high levels of IL-8 in psoriasis have also been suggested to stimulate angiogenesis [22] and keratinocyte proliferation [23]. However, neither the focal expression of IL-8 and GROα nor the expression of the corresponding receptors (CXCR1 and CXCR2) [24] support this assumption. According to the available *in situ* data, IL-8 and GROα appear to be involved in the recruitment of neutrophils. The role of IL-8 and GROα as lymphocyte attractants, as it has been demonstrated *in vitro* [25, 26], is unlikely to be relevant in psoriasis lesions because both are expressed in a pattern unrelated to the distribution of T cells (see below).

According to *in vitro* data most resident as well as passenger cells in the skin are capable of producing IL-8 and GRO upon appropriate stimulation (summarised in [27]). However, *in situ* data on expression of GROα and IL-8 in psoriasis support the concept that in the dermis GROα is selectively expressed by vessel-associated cells, whereas in the epidermis both chemokines are exclusively produced by keratinocytes and neutrophils themselves. Thus, neutrophils are now regarded as an active participant in the immunoregulatory network [28], and are an important inflammatory cell component in psoriasis because they secrete chemokines, which may even support their own recruitment. The *in vivo* data furthermore confirm the earlier *in vitro* finding that appropriately stimulated neutrophils are able to secrete IL-8 [29].

Chemokines with the ELR-motif (IL-8, GRO, ENA-78) are unlikely to be important candidates for lymphocyte recruitment in inflammatory dermatoses with lymphocyte dominance, since all lesions studied were devoid of considerable IL-8 and GRO mRNA levels (our own unpublished observations). Therefore, other chemokines which target T cell specifically may be expected to be expressed in psoriasis and other inflammatory conditions with T lymphocyte presence. We could recently demonstrate that among the T cell-attractant chemokines MCP-1, RANTES (regulated on activation, normal T cell expressed and secreted) [30], MIP-1α and β (macrophage inflammatory protein-1α and β) [31–33], IP-10 (interferon inducible protein-10) [34] and MIG (monokine induced by interferon γ) [35, 36] in particular IP-10 and MIG transcripts are selectively expressed in the upper part of the squirting papillae [37]. IP-10 immunoreactivity has been described pre-

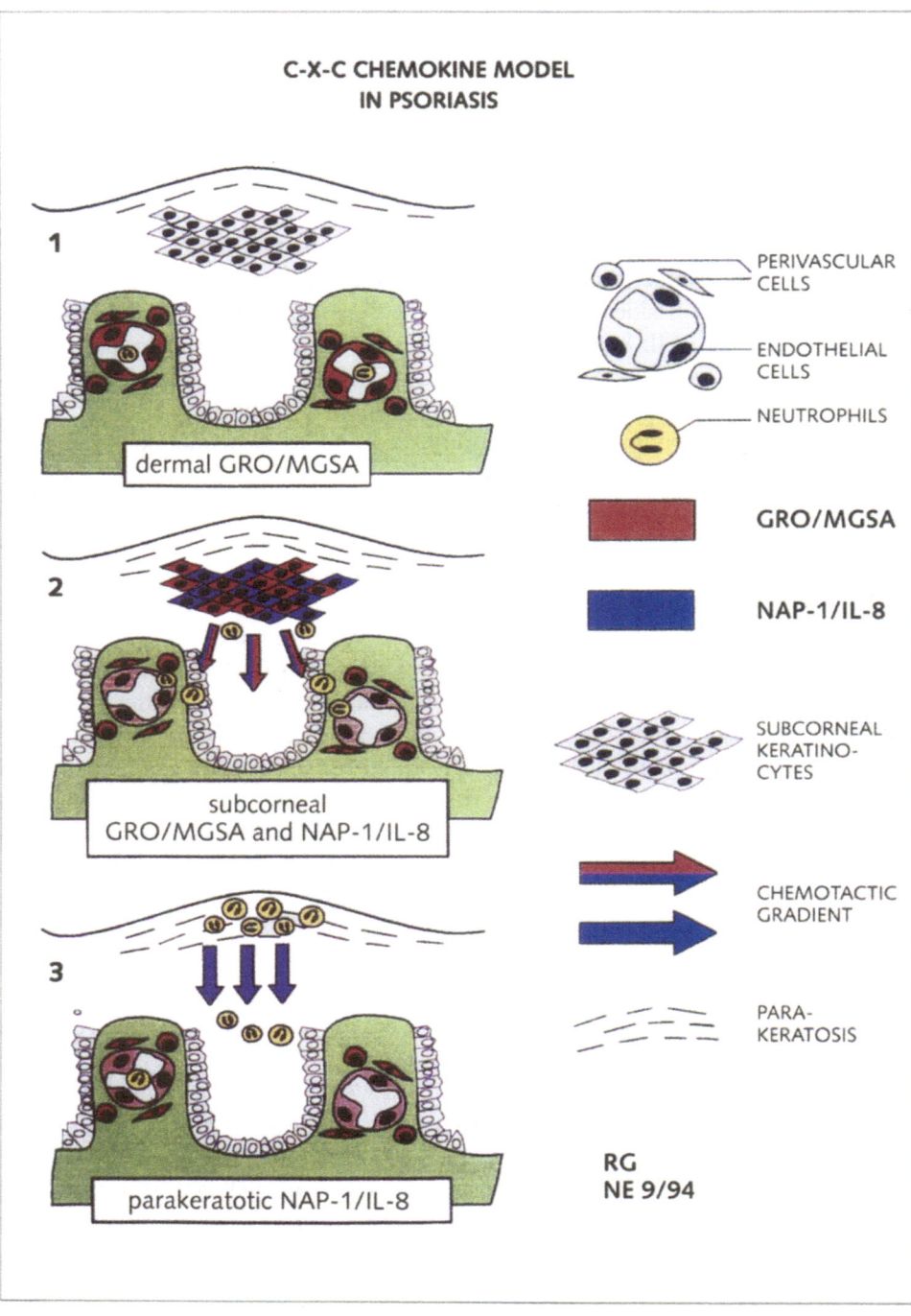

C-X-C CHEMOKINE MODEL IN PSORIASIS

1   dermal GRO/MGSA

2   subcorneal GRO/MGSA and NAP-1/IL-8

3   parakeratotic NAP-1/IL-8

PERIVASCULAR CELLS

ENDOTHELIAL CELLS

NEUTROPHILS

GRO/MGSA

NAP-1/IL-8

SUBCORNEAL KERATINO-CYTES

CHEMOTACTIC GRADIENT

PARA-KERATOSIS

RG
NE 9/94

viously [38]. However, the immunoreactivity pattern does not coincide with the mRNA expression profile [37, 38]. A similar discrepancy between the chemokine staining pattern and the distribution of the transcripts has been described for IL-8 in psoriasis [9, 10, 39, 40]. Notably, the mRNA expression is clearly spatially correlated with neutrophil infiltration, whereas a corresponding correlation has not been found using immunostaining techniques. This raises the important question as to whether chemokine immunoreactivity is a relevant parameter to assess the expression and function of chemokines *in vivo*. In the case of MIG and IP-10, the area of mRNA expression correlated with focal accumulation of T cells in the tips of the papillae. Whether other recently discovered T cell attractants are additionally involved in T cell trafficking and which factor directs T cells into the epidermal compartment remains to be elucidated. Since T cells are currently regarded as the *primum movens* in psoriasis pathology [41, 42], a detailed knowledge of lymphocyte trafficking would allow further insights into the mechanisms leading to inflammation (erythema), akanthosis and parakeratosis (scales).

As opposed to neutrophils and lymphocytes, macrophages reside in the dermis, but are frequently encountered in close contact with the basal keratinocytes of the rete ridges [43]. The distribution of these so called "lining cells" was explained by the strong expression of MCP-1 in the basal keratinocytes of psoriasis lesions [43]. *In vitro* data suggest that MCP-1 is also chemotactic for T cells [44]. The strong correlation of MCP-1 mRNA expression and co-localisation of macrophages, however, supports the notion that MCP-1 expressed by basal keratinocytes of the skin is primarily a chemoattractant for macrophages rather than for T cells.

Taken together, among the plethora of chemokines, there is a rather restricted expression of chemokines in the chronic inflammatory lesion of psoriasis: currently,

Figure 1

Model of neutrophil recruitment in psoriatic lesions

1) Initially, GRO is expressed and presented on endothelial and perivascular cells of an evolving psoriatic lesion. This, together with the expression of adhesion molecules, leads to diapedesis of neutrophils from upper dermal vessels to the papillary dermal compartment.

2) Simultaneous and co-localized focal expression of GRO and IL-8 in upper level lesional keratinocytes leads to neutrophil trafficking into the upper stratum malphighii.

3) Finally, neutrophils accumulated at the upper viable layer of the epidermis produce IL-8 themselves and thus further enhance neutrophil recruitment. Due to the epidermal turnover, neutrophils are shifted into the stratum corneum forming the typical psoriatic microabscesses.

The process of neutrophil recruitment probably takes place multifocally and periodically and may explain the different GRO and IL-8 hybridisation patterns detectable within one lesion.

IL-8, GROα, MCP-1 and MIG are clearly the dominant chemokines which are responsible for the recruitment of leukocytes such as neutrophils, macrophages and T cells. Whether such an expression profile with predominance of particular chemokines is unique for psoriasis or may also be seen in other skin diseases such as chronic eczema has to be elucidated.

Chemokines and contact hypersensitivity

Contact hypersensitivity (allergic contact dermatitis), a common inflammatory skin disease in humans, is regarded as a T cell mediated delayed hypersensitivity response. Two phases of an evolving allergic reaction have to be distinguished: (1) During the afferent or sensitisation phase epicutaneously applied antigen is processed by epidermal Langerhans cells which then migrate to the draining regional lymph nodes to present their processed antigen to naïve T cells. These T cells get primed and convert to antigen-specific memory or effector T cells. (2) In the elicitation phase the contact with small amounts of the same antigen elicits a strong inflammatory response which is hapten-specific. In addition, most allergens also display proinflammatory irritant properties which are supposed to facilitate hapten-specific immune responses (for review see [45]).

Most studies analysing chemokine expression during allergic contact dermatitis focus on their occurrence during the elicitation phase. Only a few reports refer to chemokine expression during the process of sensitisation. Enk and Katz found elevated levels of MIP-2 and IP-10 mRNA in epidermal cell extracts within 4 h after epicutaneous hapten application in non-sensitised mice [46]. Cell depletion studies suggested that both chemokines were produced by keratinocytes. Early studies employing rabbit antisera or monoclonal antibodies for immunohistochemistry demonstrated keratinocyte-associated immunoreactivity in patients with allergic contact dermatitis [47, 48]. However, as mentioned above, chemokine immunoreactivity is unreliable and neither reflects chemokine expression nor correlates with the recruitment of the corresponding targets cells. Several groups reported on the expression of chemokine mRNA during the course of allergic contact dermatitis in mice.

Gautam and colleagues employed *in situ* hybridisation to study the distribution of MCP-1 and IP-10 expression after elicitation of contact dermatitis in trini-

Figure 2
MCP-1 mRNA expression in a human normal healing wound at day 4 after injury. MCP-1 message detected with radioactive in situ *hybridisation is visible in basal keratinocytes at the previous wound margin and within the dermal inflammatory foci. The reepithelialized area (at the right) is devoid of MCP-1 specific signals. (A) bright field illumination, (B) dark field illumination.*

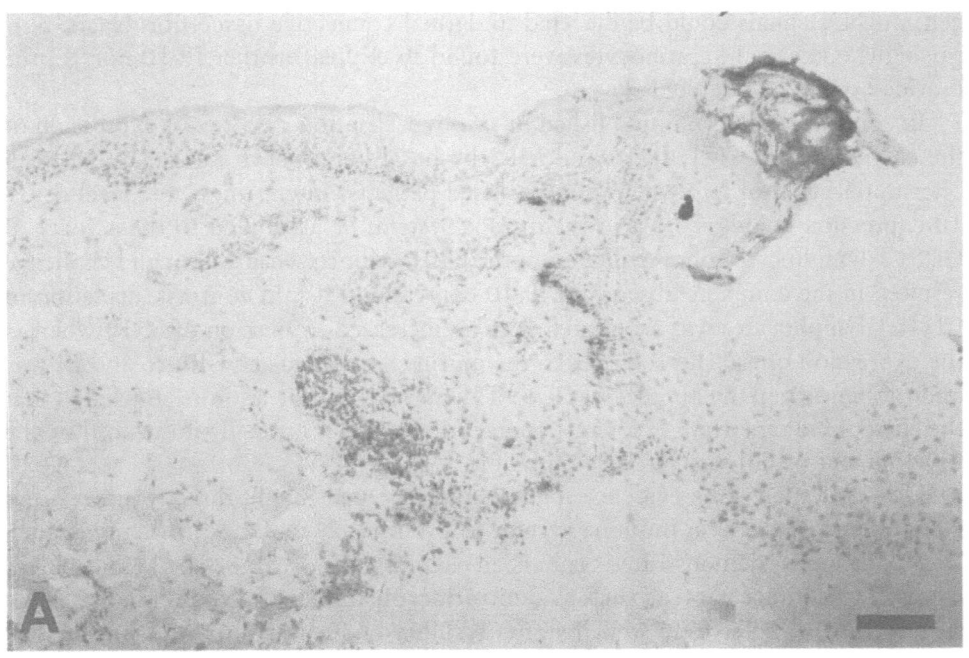

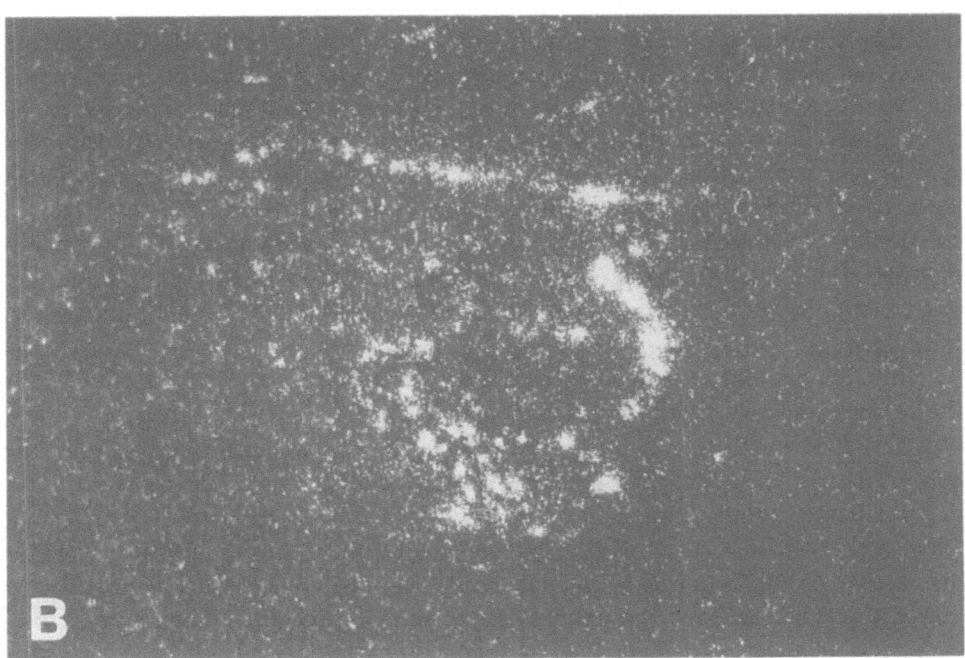

trochlorobenzene-sensitised mice [49]. As early as 4 h after application of the allergen, mRNA signals could be detected in dermal connective tissue fibroblasts. Surprisingly, epidermal keratinocytes were found to express neither IP-10 nor JE, the murine homologue of MCP-1.

In contrast, our own unpublished *in situ* hybridisation data reveal expression of the chemokines MCP-1, IP-10 and MIG by basal keratinocytes at 24 h and 48 h after application of haptens to nonsensitised patients. Interestingly, the level of IP-10 expression could, at least in the murine system, be attributed to the activity of CD8+ T lymphocytes since depletion of the latter prior to sensitisation and challenge resulted in the complete absence of IP-10 expression [50]. In contrast, depletion of CD4+ T lymphocytes was associated with an increased expression of IP-10 whereas the expression of the chemokine KC, the murine homologue of GROα, and JE was almost identical in the absence of CD4+ T lymphocytes. The authors concluded that the chemokine repertoire of allergic contact dermatitis is critically influenced by the development of different T cell populations [50].

However, increasing evidence suggests that allergens might directly affect other components of the skin immune system to produce chemokines: Mohamadzadeh and colleagues demonstrated enhanced expression of IL-8 by keratinocytes exposed to contact haptens such as dinitrofluorobenzene *in vitro*. Similarly, exposure to distinct tolerogens and irritants resulted in significant expression of IL-8 [51, 52]. Own data revealed that the metal haptens nickel and cobalt, which frequently lead to contact dermatitis in industrialised countries, are capable of not only directly inducing endothelial adhesion molecules [53] but also of enhancing expression of CC and CXC chemokines such as MCP-1, RANTES, IL-8 and GROα when exposed to isolated dermal microvascular endothelial cells [54]. These observations suggest that not only specific antigenic properties but also nonspecific proinflammatory signals delivered by haptens contribute to the chemokine pattern of allergic contact dermatitis. It is thus conceivable that certain chemokines such as MCP-1 and IL-8 may be induced by nonspecific proinflammatory hapten activities, whereas expression of others, e.g. IP-10 and MIG, are due to stimulation by cytokines released from hapten-specific T-lymphocytes, e.g. interferon γ.

Although circumstantial evidence suggests an important role of chemokines for the recruitment of leukocytes and the composition of the inflammatory infiltrate, only few functional data exist which evaluate the role of chemokines during the course of allergic contact dermatitis. So far, only data analysing the role of MCP-1 are available. Kupper and colleagues [55] studied transgenic mice which constitutively expressed murine JE/MCP-1 under the control of the human keratin 14 promoter. Despite production of high levels of functional MCP-1 by basal keratinocytes, these mice did not exhibit spontaneous cutaneous inflammation. However, when mice were sensitised to an obligate contact allergen, dinitrofluorobenzene, and challenged thereafter, significantly increased ear swelling reactions and a more pronounced mononuclear infiltrate could be observed when compared to nontransgenic mice. A recent study by Rand et al. demonstrated that application of neutralising antibodies to MCP-1 inhibited T cell and monocyte recruitment in a rat model of cutaneous delayed hypersensitivity [56]. Taken together, these observations indicate that MCP-1 appears to be functionally relevant for the pathogenesis of contact hypersensitivity reactions. Functional data regarding the role of other chemokines are still pending. Nevertheless, their spatial and temporal expression during the course of contact dermatitis which correlates well with the recruitment of distinct leukocyte subsets suggests that they are of similar importance.

Chemokine expression in other inflammatory skin disorders

Until now, chemokines have been studied in only a few inflammatory skin disorders. In localised cutaneous leishmaniasis (LCL) macrophages are an essential cell population since they are host cells for leishmania parasites, antigen presenting cells and effector cells. The high percentage of macrophages (>70% of CD45$^+$ cells) in cutaneous lesions has been explained by the strong expression of MCP-1 [57]. Surprisingly, in diffuse cutaneous leishmaniasis (DCL), a progressive and severe manifestation of cutaneous leishmaniasis with an even higher number of macrophages, MCP-1 mRNA expression is strongly reduced and compensated by the upregulated expression of MIP-1α mRNA. Since macrophages in LCL, but not in DCL, are able to intracellularly kill the parasite, MCP-1 and MIP-1α may exhibit different additional functions besides recruitment of macrophages and possibly T cells. Indeed, recent *in vitro* data demonstrate that, in contrast to MIP-1α, MCP-1 is able to stimulate the intracellular killing of parasites, indicating that different macrophage-attractant chemokines exhibit different macrophage stimulating functions (U. Ritter and H. Moll, personal communication). Moreover, it is tempting to speculate that particular chemokines are more related to a TH-1 or TH-2 immune response, respectively [58]. In LCL MCP-1 is associated with a TH-1 response (LCL) whereas in DCL MIP-1α is associated with a lack of TH-1 responsiveness. Similarly, both IP-10 and MIG appear to be highly expressed in LCL, whereas in DCL expression is significantly reduced (U. Ritter, A. Toksoy, H. Moll, R. Gillitzer, unpublished results). Since IP-10 and MIG are induced by IFNγ [34, 35], both chemokines are certainly more related to a TH-1 response. These data indicate that the dichotomy of TH-1 and TH-2 responses is not only due to the direct action of the corresponding cytokines (e.g. IL-2, IFNγ, IL-4, IL-10, IL-13). It is most likely that *in vivo* chemokines are essential mediators of these immune response patterns.

Recent unpublished data demonstrate that in interface dermatitis such as lichen planus (LP) (U. Spandau, A. Toksoy, M. Goebeler, E.B. Bröcker, R. Gillitzer, submitted) and erythema multiforme (EM) (U. Spandau, A. Toksoy, E. Kämpgen, E.B.

Bröcker, R. Gillitzer, submitted) chemokines which attract mononuclear leukocytes are selectively expressed. The microanatomic location of RANTES, MCP-1, MIP-1α and β as well as of IP-10 and MIG expression coincides with the localisation of macrophages and lymphocytes at the interface regions of both LP and EM lesions.

In skin wounds, inflammation is intimately associated with wound healing. Thereby, inflammatory cells are not only responsible for protection against local infections but are also considered to be important producers of growth factors during tissue repair. The presence of GROα and its corresponding receptor (CXCR2) in human burn wounds implicates this cytokine as an autocrine or paracrine mediator of epidermal regeneration in cutaneous wound repair [59]. In a human model of artificial wounds spatial distribution and kinetics of leukocyte immigration are correlated with the expression of IL-8, GROα, MCP-1 and MIG, suggesting an important role of particular chemokines in skin wound healing (E. Engelhardt, A. Toksoy, M. Goebeler, E.B. Bröcker, R. Gillitzer, submitted). The role of MCP-1 for macrophage recruitment has been demonstrated by DiPietro in a mouse wound healing model [60]. The similarities of the expression of chemokines in wound healing and psoriasis are striking. In both lesions, there is a focal hyperproliferation of keratinocytes and inflammation of neutrophils, macrophages and lymphocytes, albeit with different distribution and kinetics.

Taken together, these studies confirm the assumption that the distribution and composition of inflammatory cells basically reflect the chemokine expression profile. However, it remains to be answered why, despite the capacity of keratinocytes, fibroblasts, endothelial cells and inflammatory passenger cells to produce many different chemokines *in vitro*, *in vivo* chemokine expression is spatially and cellularly highly restricted.

Role of chemokines in skin tumors

In cutaneous T cell lymphoma, the epidermotropisms of neoplastic T cells into the epidermis has been explained by the epidermal presence of IL-8 and IP-10 [61-63]. Since these studies are mainly based on chemokine detection by immunohistochemistry, methods generally regarded as unreliable for reasons mentioned above, a detailed study correlating focal epidermotropism and chemokine mRNA expression is still lacking.

Figure 3
MCP-1 mRNA expression in Kaposi's sarcoma. MCP-1 transcripts visualised by radioactive in situ hybridisation (C, D) are restricted to the tumor area composed of endothelial cells. (A) immunohistological staining for CD34+ endothelial cells and CD68+ macrophages (B). (A, B, C) bright field illumination; (D) dark field illumination.

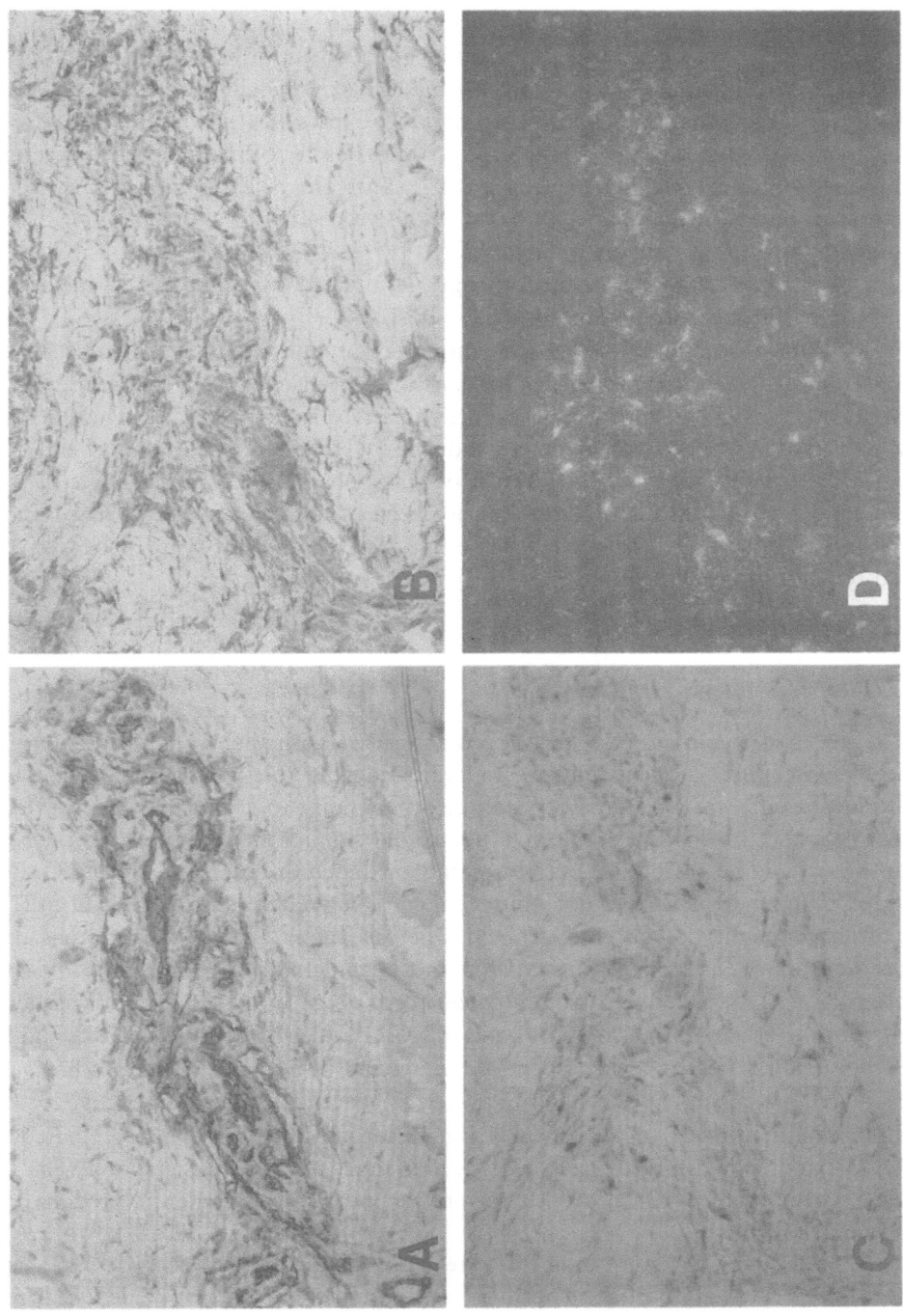

In malignant melanoma, GRO and IL-8 have been implicated as important growth factors [12, 64–66]. Since melanoma cells, at least *in vitro*, express the CXCR2 [67], basically all chemokines with the ELR-motif (e.g. IL-8, GRO, ENA-78, GCP-2 [68]) should stimulate melanoma cell growth. Thus far, a detailed study on *in vivo* localisation of CXC chemokine expression at different stages of melanoma progression and melanoma metastasis has not been published. Therefore, the question as to whether expression of IL-8 or other chemokines influence the course of human melanoma, as it has previously been suggested from *in vitro* data and animal studies, remains to be answered [67, 69, 70]. According to the data of Graves et al. recruitment of macrophages is induced by primary and metastatic melanoma through production of MCP-1 [71].

In Kaposi's sarcoma, a tumor composed of endothelial cells and dermal macrophages, the presence of macrophages has been explained by high levels of MCP-1 expressed by the spindle shaped tumor cells (Fig. 3) [72]. The question whether MCP-1 expression is directly induced by HHV-8 infection [73] of endothelial cells thus initiating the recruitment of macrophages which are capable of producing endothelial growth factors has not been completely answered. In addition, the role of potentially angiogenic chemokines as IL-8 and GRO in Kaposi's sarkoma remains to be elucidated.

Summary

The microanatomic structure of the skin together with the availability of biopsy specimens offer major advantages for evaluating the role of chemokines *in vivo*. Studies of different inflammatory skin disorders point to a selective and restricted expression of chemokines. Selective neutrophil immigration, seen in psoriasis or during wound healing, appears to be mainly mediated through IL-8 and GRO. Provided that the epidermis is not injured, there is a predominance of GRO mRNA expression in the dermal compartment whereas dermal IL-8 expression has only been encountered in open skin wounds. In the epidermis, IL-8 and GRO message are coexpressed, assuming that neutrophil recruitment in the epidermis is associated with the usage of both receptor types (CXCR1 and CXCR2). Since GRO and IL-8 expression is keratinocyte-associated, expression of both chemokines is probably regulated by a similar mechanism. Macrophage trafficking, irrespective of the inflammatory profile of a particular skin disorder, appears to be dominated by MCP-1 and, to a lesser extent, by MIP-1α (cutaneous leishmaniasis). For T cells, the CXC chemokines MIG and IP-10 currently appear to represent the predominant chemoattractants.

The selective expression of chemokines in inflammatory skin disorders indicates that *in vivo* regulation of their production is complex and cannot be deduced from *in vitro* studies. The question of downregulation or blockage of chemokine induction as a possible explanation for selectivity and restriction of chemokine expression *in vivo* has not sufficiently been addressed. In addition, determination of chemokine expression *in vivo* may also be of value to assess the progression of diseases such as melanoma. According to the currently available *in vivo* studies of skin dermatoses chemokines appear to represent the dominant factors for selective and spatial accumulation of leukocyte subsets. This nourishes thoughts for local therapeutical strategies to selectively block the recruitment of disease-promoting leukocytes using chemokine antagonists as recently described in HIV research.

References

1   Schröder JM, Christophers E (1986) Identification of C5a des arg and an anionic neutrophil-activating peptide (ANAP) in psoriatic scales. *J Invest Dermatol* 87: 53–58

2   Schröder JM, Mrowietz U, Morita U, Christophers E (1987) Purification and partial biochemical characterization of a human monocyte-derived neutrophil-activating peptide that lacks interleukin 1 activity. *J Immunol* 139: 3474–3483

3   Yoshimura T, Matsushima K, Tanaka S, Robinson EA, Appella E, Oppenheim JJ, Leonard EJ (1987) Purification of a human monocyte-derived neutrophil chemotactic factor that shares sequence homology with other host defense cytokines. *Proc Natl Acad Sci USA* 84: 9233–9238

4   Walz A, Peveri P, Aschauer AO, Baggiolini M (1987) Purification and amino acid sequencing of NAF, a novel neutrophil activating factor produced by monocytes. *Biochem Biophys Res Commun* 149: 755–761

5   Matsushima K, Morishita K, Yoshimura T, Lavu S, Kobayashi Y, Lew W, Appella E, Kung HF, Leonard EJ, Oppenheim JJ (1988) Molecular cloning of a human monocyte-derived neutrophil chemotactic factor (MDNCF) and the induction of tumor necrosis factor. *J Exp Med* 167: 1833–1893

6   Yoshimura T, Robinson EA, Tanaka S, Appella E, Kuratsu J, Leonard EJ (1989) Purification and amino acid analysis of two glioma-derived monocyte chemoattractants. *J Exp Med* 169: 1449–1459

7   Matsushima K, Larsen CG, DuBois GC, Oppenheim JJ (1989) Purification and characterization of a novel monocyte chemotactic and activating factor produced by a human myelomonocytic cell line. *J Exp Med* 169: 1485–1490

8   Gillitzer R, Berger R, Mielke V, Müller C, Wolff K, Stingl G (1991) Upper keratinocytes of psoriatic skin lesions express high levels of NAP-1/IL-8 mRNA *in situ*. *J Invest Dermatol* 97: 73–79

9   Gillitzer R, Ritter U, Spandau U, Goebeler M, Bröcker EB (1996). Differential expression of GRO-α and IL-8 mRNA in psoriasis: a model for neutrophil migration and accumulation *in vivo*. *J Invest Dermatol* 107: 778–782

10   Kulke R, Tödt-Pingel I, Rademacher D, Röwert J, Schröder JM, Christophers E (1996) Co-localized overexpression of GRO-α and IL-8 mRNA is restricted to the suprapapillary layers of psoriatic lesions. *J Invest Dermatol* 106: 526–530

11   Anisowicz A, Bardwell L, Sager R (1987) Constitutive overexpression of a growth-regulated gene in transformed Chinese hamster and human cells. *Proc Natl Acad Sci USA* 84: 7188–7192

12   Richmond A, Balentien E, Thomas HG, Flaggs G, Barton DE, Spiess J, Bordoni R, Francke U, Derynck R (1988) Molecular characterization and chromosomal mapping of melanoma growth stimulatory activity, a growth factor structurally related to β-thromboglobulin. *EMBO J* 7: 2025–2033

13   Walz A, Burgener R, Car B, Baggiolini M, Kunkel SL, Strieter RM (1991) Structure and neutrophil-activating properties of a novel inflammatory peptide (ENA-78) with homology to interleukin 8. *J Exp Med* 174: 1355–1362

14   Kojima T, Cromie MA, Fisher GJ, Voorhees JJ, Elder JT (1993) Gro-α mRNA is selectively overexpressed in psoriatic epidermis and is reduced by Cyclosporin A *in vivo*, but not in cultured keratinocytes. *J Invest Dermatol* 101: 767–772

15   Springer TA (1994) Traffic signals for leukocyte circulation. *Cell* 76: 301–314

16   Goebeler M, Yoshimura T, Toksoy A, Ritter U, Bröcker EB, Gillitzer R (1997) The chemokine repertoire of human microvascular endothelial cells and its regulation by inflammatory cytokines. *J Invest Dermatol* 107: 778–782

17   Rot A, Hub E, Middleton J, Pons F, Rabeck C, Thierer K, Wintle J, Wolff B, Zsak M, Dukor P (1996) Some aspects of IL-8 pathophysiology III: chemokine interaction with endothelial cells. *J Leukoc Biol* 59: 39–44

18   Murphy PM, Tiffany HL (1991) Cloning of complementary DNA encoding a functional human interleukin-8 receptor. *Science* 253: 1280–1283

19   Holms WE, Lee J, Kuang WJ, Rice GC, Wood WI (1991) Structure and functional expression of a human interleukin-8 receptor. *Science* 253: 1278–1280

20   Lee J, Horuk R, Rice GC, Bennett GL, Camerato T, Wood WI (1992) Characterization of two high affinity human interleukin-8 receptors. *J Biol Chem* 267: 16283–16287

21   Herbert CA, Lowman HB (1996) Structure-function relationship of IL-8 and its two neutrophil receptors: IL-8RA and IL-8RB. In: Horuk R (ed): *Chemoattractant ligands and their receptors.* CRC Press, Boca Raton, 29–53

22   Nickoloff BJ, Mitra RS, Varani J, Dixit VM, Polverini PJ (1994) Aberrant production of interleukin-8 and thrombospondin-1 by psoriatic keratinocytes mediates angiogenesis. *Am J Pathol* 144: 820–828

23   Tuschil AC, Lam C, Halsberger A, Lindley I (1992) Interleukin-8 stimulates calcium transients and promotes epidermal cell proliferation. *J Invest Dermatol* 99: 294–298

24   Bornscheuer E, Schröder JM, Christophers M,E, Sticherling M (1997) Psoriatic keratinocytes express the interleukin 8 receptor B. *Arch Dermatol Res* 289: A57

25   Larsen CG, Anderson OA, Oppenheim JJ, Matsushima K (1989) Neutrophil activating protein (NAP-1) is also chemotactic for T lymphocytes. *Science* 243: 1464–1466

26 Jinquan T, Frydenberg J, Mukaida N, Bonde J, Larsen CG, Matsushima K, Thestrup-Pedersen K (1995) Recombinant human growth-related oncogene-α induces T lymphocyte chemotaxis. *J Immunol* 155: 5359–5368

27 Vaddi K, Keller M, Newton RC (eds) (1996) *The chemokine facts book*. Academic Press, San Diego

28 Lloyd AR, Oppenheim JJ (1992) Poly's lament: the neglected role of the polymorphnuclear neutrophil in the afferent limb of the immune system. *Immunol Today* 13: 169–171

29 Bazzoni F, Cassatella MA, Rossi F, Ceska M, Dewald B, Baggiolini M (1991) Phagocytosing neutrophils produce and release high amounts of the neutrophil-activating peptide/interleukin 8. *J Exp Med* 173: 771–774

30 Schall JT, Bacon K, Toy KJ, Goeddel DV (1990) Selective attraction of monocytes and T lymphocytes of the memory phenotype by cytokine RANTES. *Nature* 347: 669–671

31 Wolpe SD, Davatelis G, Sherry B, Beutler B, Hesse DG, Nguyen HT, Moldawer LL, Nathan CF, Lowry SF, Cerami A (1988) Macrophages secrete a novel heparin-binding protein with inflammatory and neutrophil chemokinetic properties. *J Exp Med* 167: 570–581

32 Sherry B, Tecamp-Olson P, Gallegos C, Bauer D, Davatelis G, Wolpe SD, Masiarz F, Coit D, Cerami A (1988) Resolution of the two components of macrophage inflammatory protein-1, and cloning and characterization of one of the components, macrophage inflammatory protein 1β. *J Exp Med* 168: 2251–2259

33 Schall JT, Bacon K, Camp RD, Kaspari JW, Goeddel DV (1993) Human macrophage inflammatory protein-α (MIP-1α) and MIP-1β chemokines attract distinct populations of lymphocytes. *J Exp Med* 77: 1821–1826

34 Luster AD and Ravetch JV (1987) Genomic characterization of a g-interferon-inducible gene (IP-10) and identification of an interferon-inducible hypersensitive site. *Mol Cell Biol* 7: 3723–3731.

35 Faber JM (1993) HuMIG: a new member of the chemokine family of cytokines. *Biochem Biophys Res Commun* 192: 223–230.

36 Liao F, Rabin RL, Yannelli JR, Konoriaris LG, Vanguri P, Farber JM (1995) Human MIG chemokine: biochemical and functional characterization. *J Exp Med* 182: 1301–1337.

37 Goebeler M, Toksoy A, Spandau U, Bröcker EB, Gillitzer R (1998) MIG chemokine is highly expressed in the papillae of psoriatic lesions. *J Pathol* 184: 89–95

38 Gottlieb AB, Luster AD, Posnett DN, Carter DM (1988) Detection of a γ-interferon-induced protein IP-10 in psoriatic plaques. *J Exp Med* 168: 941–948

39 Sticherling M, Bornscheuer E, Schröder JM, Christophers E (1991) Localization of neutrophil-activating peptide-1/interleukin-8 immunoreactivity in normal and psoriatic skin. *J Invest Dermatol* 96: 26–30

40 Antilla HSI, Reitamo S, Erkko P, Ceska M, Moser B, Baggiolini M (1992) Interleukin-8 immunoreactivity of healthy subjects and patients with palmoplantar pustulosis and psoriasis. *J Invest Dermatol* 98: 96–101

41 Gottlieb SL, Gilleaudeau P, Johnson R, Estes L, Woodworth TG, Gottlieb AB, Krueger JG (1995) Response of psoriasis to a lymphocyte-selective toxin (DAB389IL-2) suggests a primary immune, but not keratinocyte, pathogenic basis. *Nature Med* 1: 442–447

42 Schön MP, Detmar M, Parker CM (1997) Murine psoriasis-like disorder induced by naive CD4+ T cells. *Nature Med* 3: 183–189

43 Gillitzer R, Wolff K, Tong D, Müller Ch, Yoshimura T, Hartmann AA, Stingl G, Berger R (1993) MCP-1 mRNA expression in basal keratinocytes of psoriatic lesions. *J Invest Dermatol* 101: 127–131

44 Taub DD, Proost P, Murphy WJ, Anver M, Longo DL, van Damme J, Oppenheim JJ (1995) Monocyte chemotactic proteins-1 (MCP-1), -2, and -3 are chemotactic for human T-lymphocytes. *J Clin Invest* 95: 1370–1376

45 Grabbe S, Schwarz T (1996) Immunoregulatory mechanisms involved in elicitation of allergic contact hypersensitivity. *Am J Contact Derm* 7: 238–246

46 Enk AH, Katz SI (1992) Early molecular events in the induction phase of contact sensitivity. *Proc Natl Acad Sci USA* 89: 1389–1402

47 Griffiths CEM, Barker JNWN, Kunkel S, Nickoloff BJ (1991) Modulation of leucocyte adhesion molecules, a T cell chemotaxin (IL-8) and a regulatory cytokine (TNF-α) in allergic contact dermatitis (rhus dermatitis). *Brit J Dermatol* 124: 519–526

48. Sticherling M, Bornscheuer E, Schröder JM, Christophers E (1992) Immunohistochemical studies on NAP-1/IL-8 in contact eczema and atopic dermatitis. *Arch Dermatol Res* 284: 82–85

49. Gautam S, Battisto J, Major JA, Amstrong D, Stoler M, Hamilton TA (1994) Chemokine expression in trinitrochlorobenzene-mediated contact hypersensitivity. *J Leukoc Biol* 55: 452–460

50 Abe M, Kondo T, Xu H, Fairchild RL (1996) Interferon-γ inducible protein (IP-10) expression is mediated by CD8+ T cells and is regulated by CD4+ T cells during elicitation of contact hypersensitivity. *J Invest Dermatol* 107: 360–366

51 Mohamadzadeh M, Müller M, Hultsch T, Enk A, Saloga J, Knop J (1994) Enhanced expression of IL-8 in normal human keratinocytes and human keratinocyte cell line HaCaT *in vitro* after stimulation with contact sensitizers, tolerogens and irritants. Exp Dermatol 3: 298–303

52 Wilmer JL, Burleson FG, Kayama F, Kanno J, Luster MI (1994) Cytokine induction in human epidermal keratinocytes exposed to contact irritants and its relation to chemical-induced inflammation in mouse skin. *J Invest Dermatol* 102: 915–922

53 Goebeler M, Meinardus-Hager G, Roth J, Goerdt S, Sorg C (1993) Nickel chloride and cobalt chloride, two common contact sensitizers, directly induce expression of ICAM-1, VCAM-1 and ELAM-1 by endothelial cells. *J Invest Dermatol* 100: 759–765

54 Goebeler M, Ritter U, Toksoy A, Binder R, Bröcker EB, Werner S, Yoshimura T, Schulze-Osthoff K, Gillitzer R (1995) Nickel and cobalt, two common haptens leading to contact allergy, directly induce endothelial expression of CC- and CXC-chemokines. Fourth International Chemokine Symposium "Molecules to Disease", Bath UK, p. 11

55 Nakamura K, Williams IR, Kupper TS (1995) Keratinocyte-derived monocyte chemoat-

tractant protein-1 (MCP-1): Analysis in a transgenic model demonstrates MCP-1 can recruit dendritic and Langerhans cells to skin. *J Invest Dermatol* 105: 633–643

56 Rand M, Warren JS, Mansour MK, Newman W, Ringler DJ (1996) Inhibition of T cell recruitment and cutaneous delayed-type hypersensitivity-induced inflammation with antibodies to monocyte chemoattractant protein-1. *Am J Pathol* 148: 855–864

57 Ritter U, Moll H, Laskay T, Bröcker EB, Velazco O, Becker I, Gillitzer R (1996) Differential expression of chemokines in patients with localized and diffuse cutaneous American leishmaniasis. *J Infect Dis* 173: 699–709

58 Mosmann TR, Cherwinski H, Bond MW, Giedlin MA, Coffman RL (1986) Two types of murine T helper cell clones. I. Definition according to profiles of lymphokine activities and secreted proteins. *J Immunol* 136: 2348–2357

59 Nanney LB, Mueller SG, Bueno R, Peiper SC, Richmond A (1995) Distributions of melanoma growth stimulatory activity or growth-regulated gene and the interleukin-8 receptor B in human wound repair. *Am J Pathol* 147: 1248–1260

60 DiPietro LA, Polverini PJ, Rahbe SM, Kovacs EJ (1995) Modulation of JE/MCP-1 expression in dermal wound repair. *Am J Pathol* 146: 868–875

61 Hansen ER, Vejlsgaard GL, Lisby S, Heidenheim M, Baadsgaard O (1991) Epidermal interleukin-1α functional activity and interleukin-8 immunoreactivity are increased in patients with cutaneous T cell lymphoma. *J Invest Dermatol* 97: 818–823

62 McLean Wismer J, McKenzie RC, Sauder DN (1994) Interleukin-8 immunoreactivity in epidermis of cutaneous T cell lymphoma patients. *Lymphokine Cytokine Res* 13: 21–27

63 Sarris AH, Esgleyes-Ribot T, Crow M, Broxmeyer HE, Karasavvas N, Pugh W, Grossman D, Deisseroth A, Duvic M (1995) Cytokine loops involving interferon-γ and IP-10, a cytokine chemotactic for CD4+ lymphocytes: an explanation for the epidermotropism of cutaneous T cell lymphoma. *Blood* 86: 651–658

64 Richmond A, Thomas HG (1988) Melanoma growth stimulating activity: isolation from human melanoma tumors and characterization of tissue distribution. *J Cell Biochem* 36: 185–192

65 Schadendorf D, Möller A, Algermissen B, Worm M, Sticherling M, Czarnetzki BM (1993) IL-8 produced by human malignant melanoma cells *in vitro* is an essential autocrine growth factor. *J Immunol* 151: 2667–2675

66 Singh RK, Gutman M, Radinsky R, Bucana CD, Fidler IJ (1994) Expression of interleukin-8 correlates with the metastatic potential of human melanoma cells in nude mice. *Cancer Res* 54: 3242–3247

67 Norgauer J, Metzner B, Schraufstätter I (1996) Expression and growth promoting functions of the IL-8 receptor β in human melanoma cells. *J Immunol* 156: 1132–1137

68 Rovai LE, Hershman HR, Smith JB (1997) Cloning and characterization of the human granulocyte chemotactic protein-2 gene. *J Immunol* 158: 5257–5266

69 Hayashi S, Kurdowska A, Cohen AB, Stevens MD, Fujisawa N, Miller EJ (1997) A synthetic peptide inhibitor for α-chemokines inhibits the growth of melanoma cell lines. *J Clin Invest* 99: 2581–2587

70 Singh RK, Gutman M, Reich R, Bar-Eli M (1995) Ultraviolet B irradiation promotes tumorigenic and metastatic properties in primary cutaneous melanoma via induction of interleukin 8. *Cancer Res* 55: 3699–3674

71 Graves DT, Barnhill R, Galanopoulos T, Antionades HN (1992) Expression of monocyte chemoattractant protein-1 in human melanoma *in vivo. Am J Pathol* 140: 9–14

72 Gillitzer R, Berger R (1991) High levels of macrophage chemotactic protein-1 and interleukin-6 in lesions of Kaposi's Sarcoma *in situ. J Cell Biochem Suppl* 15F: 249

73 Chang Y, Cesarman E, Pessin MS, Lee F, Culpepper J, Knowless DM, Morre PS (1994) Identification of Herpesvirus-like DANN sequences in AIDS-associated Kaposi's sarcoma. *Science* 266: 1865–1869

Index